Probing Selected Autoimmune Diseases for Focused Perspectives

Edited by Mourad Aribi

Published in London, United Kingdom

Probing Selected Autoimmune Diseases for Focused Perspectives
http://dx.doi.org/10.5772/intechopen.1000271
Edited by Mourad Aribi

Contributors
Ailan Zhao, Elena Klimova, Guimei Cai, Huanhuan Yang, Jingping Cai, Larisa Drozdova, Maynor Herrera-Méndez, Mourad Aribi, Nurakant Neupane, Olena Lavinska, Ping Zheng, Qiuping Fan, Sergey Sushkov, Valery Boyko, WanChao Wang, Xiaojing Nie, Yi Chen, Yuanzhen Zhang, Yueting Gong, Yunfan Zhang, Yuxian Tang, Zihan Dai

First published in London, United Kingdom, 2024 by IntechOpen
IntechOpen is the global imprint of INTECHOPEN LIMITED, registered in England and Wales, registration number: 11086078, 5 Princes Gate Court, London, SW7 2QJ, United Kingdom

British Library Cataloguing-in-Publication Data
A catalogue record for this book is available from the British Library

Additional hard and PDF copies can be obtained from orders@intechopen.com

Probing Selected Autoimmune Diseases for Focused Perspectives
Edited by Mourad Aribi
p. cm.
Print ISBN 978-1-83769-688-8
Online ISBN 978-1-83769-687-1
eBook (PDF) ISBN 978-1-83769-689-5

For EU product safety concerns:
IN TECH d.o.o., Prolaz Marije Krucifikse Kozulić 3, 51000 Rijeka, Croatia,
info@intechopen.com or visit our website at intechopen.com.

Meet the editor

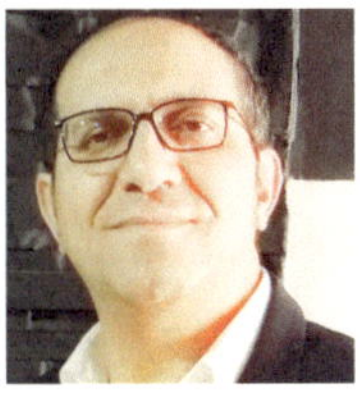

Dr. Mourad Aribi, Ph.D., Dr. Hab., Ther Immunol., HDR from the University of Montpellier, France is a Distinguished Professor of Immunology at the University of Tlemcen, Algeria. With a remarkable vision, he founded and led the Laboratory of Applied Molecular Biology and Immunology (W0414100). Additionally, he played a key role in introducing bachelor's, master's, and doctoral degrees in immunology at the University of Tlemcen. Dr. Aribi's research endeavors revolve around exploring the modulation of cell-mediated and inflammatory immune responses in autoimmune diseases, cancer, and infectious diseases. Thanks to his interdisciplinary skills, he was able to forge strong collaborations with esteemed institutions worldwide. He has successfully led numerous high-level bilateral and multilateral projects, collaborating with esteemed partners, in particular with partners from CNRS and INSERM (Montpellier, Marseille, Burgundy-Franche-Comté [France]), partners from the Institute for Immunodeficiency (Freibourg [Germany]), and, more recently, partners from Valencia University (Spain, CIBERER, Institute of Health Carlos III), Harvard Medical School (Boston, USA), and Guangdong Provincial People's Hospital (China). Dr. Aribi's immense contributions extend beyond his research, as he actively contributes to the scientific community. He serves as a valued reviewer for various international scientific journals and holds a significant position as an editorial board member of Frontiers in Immunology, the official journal of the International Union of Immunological Societies (IUIS). Through these roles, he continues to make meaningful contributions to the dissemination and advancement of scientific knowledge and continues to inspire and drive progress in immunological research and its applications for the benefit of society.

Contents

Preface

This book addresses selected autoimmune diseases, providing focused insights into their intricate landscapes. Each chapter explores specific aspects, from the delicate balance between immune tolerance and defense to the nuanced triggers of autoimmune reactions. With a pedagogic aim, this collective work offers targeted perspectives on diseases like myasthenia gravis, hepatosplenomegaly, autoimmune rheumatic diseases, Buerger's disease, and autoimmune thyroid diseases. With six chapters in total, the book aims to enhance understanding, paving the way for future research and personalized therapeutic strategies within the realm of autoimmune disorders.

Chapter 1 provides a concise and targeted overview of autoimmune diseases, highlighting the delicate balance between immune tolerance and immune defense, the regulatory mechanisms of T cells and B cells, and the complexity of these diseases. It is designed for a brief and focused understanding in a pedagogic and academic context.

Chapter 2 explores the pivotal role of intestinal mucosal immunity in autoimmune diseases, detailing its history, composition, and involvement in some conditions, including systemic lupus erythematosus, inflammatory bowel diseases, and type 1 diabetes. It also discusses progress in treating autoimmune diseases through interventions aimed at enhancing this aspect of the immune system.

In Chapter 3, the focus shifts to unveiling triggers and predictors of autoimmune reactions in myasthenia gravis and hepatosplenomegaly. Highlighting specific markers for personalized treatment, it emphasizes unique aspects in thymus-independent myasthenia gravis, splenomegaly, and genetically determined orphan storage diseases.

Chapter 4 explores mortality in autoimmune rheumatic diseases, updating concepts, highlighting geographic variations, and emphasizing the significance of measuring standardized mortality rates. It delves into causes of death, associations with acute events, and factors influencing mortality, concluding with a focus on the diverse risk landscape among such disorders.

Chapter 5 explores Buerger's disease, unraveling its autoimmune nature marked by hypersensitivity reactions. Covering clinical aspects, diagnostic criteria, and influential factors, it provides insights for diagnosis and treatment, paving the way for future research and therapeutic advancements.

Finally, in Chapter 6, attention turns to the immune system's involvement in autoimmune thyroid diseases, specifically autoimmune thyroiditis. Emphasizing the significance of anti-thyroperoxidase antibodies in both diagnosis and prognosis, the chapter outlines the research methods used for comprehensive exploration.

I genuinely hope that this book becomes a valuable resource and pedagogical aid for clinicians, researchers, basic scientists, and professionals specializing in immunology and immunopathology. It is also tailored for advanced biology and medical students, offering insights applicable to clinical practice and applied medical disciplines.

I would like to extend my sincere gratitude to all collaborators who contributed significantly to the creation of this book. My heartfelt appreciation also goes to the Publishing Process Manager and the dedicated team at IntechOpen for their trust, patience, and invaluable support throughout the publication process.

Mourad Aribi
Professor,
Laboratory of Applied Molecular Biology and Immunology,
University of Tlemcen,
Tlemcen, Algeria

Chapter 1

Introductory Chapter: Navigating Autoimmunity – From Molecular Mechanisms to Therapeutic Horizons

Mourad Aribi

1. Introduction

Autoimmune diseases, significant challenges to global health, result from immune responses targeting self-antigens [1]. Understanding these diseases requires exploring the underlying molecular mechanisms, offering crucial perspectives on targeted therapy development.

2. Balancing immunity: tolerance and defense

The immune system aims to maintain cellular and tissue integrity, reject foreign entities, and tolerate self-antigens [2, 3]. This delicate balance relies on distinguishing nonself (pathogens) and modified self-components from unmodified self-antigens, which are tolerated.

3. Key features of innate and adaptive immunity

Innate and adaptive immunity are crucial for maintaining immune system integrity. Innate immunity acts as a first line of immune defense, while adaptive immunity provides immunological memory. This feature might similarly apply to innate immunity, albeit in a distinctive manner without clonal distribution. In this regard, it's important to mention that we are presently exploring the concept of trained immunity.

4. Orchestrating tolerance: comprehensive insights into T-cell regulation and research in therapeutic potentials

T-cells under the orchestration of various regulatory mechanisms are pivotal in maintaining immunological tolerance [4]. This orchestration extends from the central tolerance mechanisms within the thymus that eliminate autoreactive T-cells [5] to peripheral tolerance mechanisms that prevent T-cell responses to self-antigens in peripheral tissues.

IntechOpen

In the periphery, mature lymphocytes navigate through a sophisticated process of encountering self-antigens, leading to intrinsic anergy, apoptosis, or regulatory control by regulatory T-cells (Tregs) [6–8]. This complex ballet of peripheral tolerance is essential in curbing T-cell responses to self-antigens.

The fate of naive T-cells is intricately influenced by the balance between antigen (Signal 1) and co-stimulation (Signal 2). Co-stimulation mediated by immune checkpoints, such as cytotoxic T-lymphocyte antigen 4 (CTLA-4) and programmed cell death protein 1 (PD-1), plays a crucial role in regulating T-cell activation [9]. Anergy in T-cells encountering self-antigens emerges from inadequate co-stimulation, involving aberrant T-cell receptor (TCR) signaling and heightened co-inhibitory signals [10, 11].

The orchestration of immune balance extends to the interplay between activating receptors (TCR complex, CD28) and inhibitory receptors (CTLA-4, PD-1). CTLA-4 halts T-cell activation by removing B7 (CD80/CD86) ligands from antigen-presenting cells (APCs), while PD-1 inhibits T-cell activation through downstream signaling [12–14]. Recognition of self-antigens induces apoptosis in T-cells through multiple mechanisms [15, 16].

This comprehensive understanding of T-cell regulation provides insights into the intricate mechanisms that maintain immunological equilibrium.

One such approach involves unleashing the immune arsenal by targeting inhibitory receptors like CTLA-4 and PD-1 in therapies. While this amplifies antitumor immune responses, it may also pose the risk of triggering autoimmune reactions. Ongoing research delves into the exploration of other inhibitory receptors as potential targets for checkpoint blockade therapy. Another avenue involves tapping into Treg cells, which play a vital role in immune balance. Treg cells suppress harmful lymphocytes through different mechanisms, including cytokine production (IL-10, TGF-β) and expression of inhibitory molecules, such as CTLA-4. Treg cell therapy is gaining traction for addressing autoimmune diseases, graft-versus-host reactions, and graft rejection. Additionally, ongoing trials are investigating the potential of IL-2 in regulating immune reactions and highlighting the therapeutic applications of Treg cells [17].

5. B-cell tolerance

Balancing B-cell tolerance is a multifaceted process crucial for immune homeostasis. During B-cell development, negative selection eliminates cells with high self-antigen affinity, preventing the production of autoantibodies. Positive selection evaluates receptor functionality with a moderate self-antigen response, while excessive self-reactivity triggers receptor reformatting, known as receptor editing, involving gene rearrangements in the immunoglobulin M (IgM) light chain loci [18].

Self-reactive B-cell tolerance mechanisms encompass various strategies, including receptor editing, deletion, anergy, and competition for growth factors. Anergy renders B-cells functionally incapacitated, particularly when recognizing soluble proteins with low avidity in the bone marrow or specific microenvironments [19].

Similar to T-cells, B-cells also undergo two types of tolerance mechanisms–central and peripheral. Central tolerance of B-cells occurs during development in the bone marrow and involves receptor editing or negative selection, targeting B-cells with high-affinity receptors for prevalent autoantigens [20]. In peripheral lymphoid tissues, mature B-cells may undergo anergy, becoming unresponsive to autoantigens independently of T-cell assistance [21]. While essential for thymus-independent self-antigens such as polysaccharides and lipids, these anergic B-cells exit lymphoid follicles, but their survival may be compromised without essential stimuli.

Loss of B-cell anergy is a pivotal aspect of the intricate B-cell tolerance mechanism. In the periphery, 20% of B-cells express self-reactive receptors, restrained by inhibitory signals that are swiftly reversed upon dissociation from self-antigens. The loss of B-cell anergy precedes selected autoimmune disorders, highlighting its potential contributions to pathogenic B-cells in autoimmunity [22]. This delicate balance is further influenced by the regulatory roles of Tregs and regulatory B cells (Bregs), contributing to immune equilibrium by curbing excessive inflammatory responses [23, 24].

6. Microbiome and fetal antigen tolerance

6.1 Microbial harmony: essential roles in immune tolerance

Commensal microbes in the gut, respiratory tract, and skin perform vital functions. Mature lymphocytes recognize microbes without triggering immune responses, aided by some mechanisms like the regulation exerted by IL-10-producing Treg cells. Intestinal dendritic cells (DCs) contribute to food antigen tolerance [25–27].

6.2 Treg cells in pregnancy

6.2.1 Orchestrating fetal antigen tolerance

Tolerance to fetal antigens during pregnancy avoids immune responses against paternal antigens. Peripheral transcription factor forkhead box protein 3 (FoxP3, also known as scurfin) specific to paternal antigens play a crucial role in immune suppression, modulating various mechanisms for fetal tolerance. Treg cells peak during trophoblast invasion, decreasing during labor, highlighting their dynamic role throughout pregnancy [28, 29].

6.2.2 Mechanisms of fetal antigen tolerance

Treg cells influence cytokines and immunological signals, excluding inflammatory cells from the uterus, and establishing an immunosuppressive placental microenvironment. Disruptions in these mechanisms may lead to immune complications during pregnancy [30, 31].

7. Autoimmunity: genetic and environmental influences

Autoimmunity emerges as a consequence of the immune system's aberrant overactivation targeting its own unaltered components. This phenomenon involves a combination of genetic predisposition, epigenetic changes, and various environmental influences, such as infections, ultraviolet (UV) radiation, medications, vaccination, and sex hormones. These factors, as depicted in **Figure 1**, interact intricately to impact disease susceptibility, prompting activation of self-reactive T-cells and B-cells. The orchestration of T-cells, B-cells, APCs, antibodies, inflammatory cells, and cytokines intricately contributes to the complexity of the autoimmune process [1].

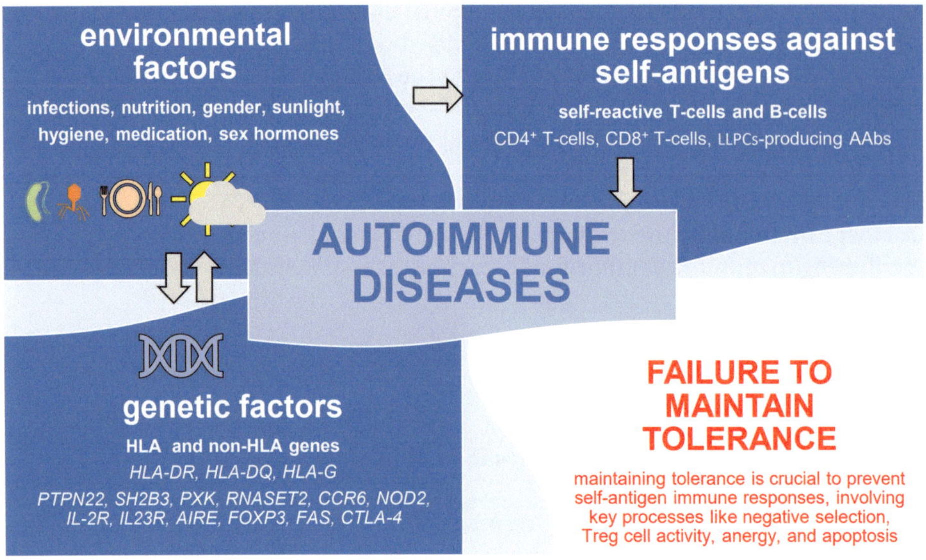

Figure 1.
Interplay of genetic and environmental factors in autoimmune diseases. This figure provides a succinct visual overview of the complex interrelationships driving autoimmune diseases. Genetic factors include variants of the HLA and non-HLA genes. Environmental factors encompass mainly infections, nutrition, gender, low sunlight (ultraviolet rays) exposure, hygiene, medications, and sex hormones. Immune responses against self-antigens involve CD4⁺ T-cells, CD8⁺ T-cells, and B-cells, as well as long-lived "memory" plasma cells producing autoantibodies. The failure to maintain tolerance, governed by key mechanisms such as negative selection, Treg cells, anergy, and apoptosis, is pivotal in understanding autoimmune disease development. These intricate interactions contribute to the development of autoimmune diseases. AIRE: Autoimmune regulator, CCR6: C-C motif chemokine receptor 6, CTLA-4: Cytotoxic T-lymphocyte antigen 4, FAS: FAS cell surface death receptor (also known as tumor necrosis factor [TNF] receptor superfamily member cluster of differentiation 95 [CD95] or apoptosis antigen 1 [APO-1 or APT]), FOXP3: Transcription factor forkhead box protein 3, HLA: Human leukocyte antigen, IL23R: Interleukin-23 receptor, IL-2R: Interleukin-2 receptor, LLPCs: Long-lived plasma cells, NOD2: Nucleotide-binding oligomerization domain-containing protein 2, PTPN22: Protein tyrosine phosphatase non-receptor type 22, RNASET2: Ribonuclease T2, SH2B3: SH2B adaptor protein 3 (also referred to as lymphocyte adapter protein [Lnk]), PXK: Phox (PX) domain-containing serine/threonine kinase.

7.1 Genetic factors

7.1.1 Role of MHC alleles

Human leukocyte antigen (HLA) alleles, particularly class II (HLA-DR and HLA-DQ), modulate immune responses involving autoreactive $CD4^+$ T-cells. Specific HLA alleles increase autoimmune disease risk, with their exact role remaining elusive. Non-classical HLA-G gene, especially soluble HLA-G (sHLA-G), is crucial for immune tolerance at the maternal-fetal interface [32–36].

7.1.2 Non-HLA genes

A myriad of non-HLA genes actively contribute to the complex landscape of autoimmune diseases, introducing polymorphisms that disrupt self-tolerance or set off abnormal lymphocyte activation. Noteworthy genes implicated in various autoimmune conditions include protein tyrosine phosphatase non-receptor type 22 (*PTPN22*), SH2B adaptor protein 3 (*SH2B3*), phox (PX) domain-containing serine/threonine kinase (*PXK*), ribonuclease T2 (*RNASET2*), and C-C motif chemokine receptor 6 (*CCR6*), among others, revealing the genetic diversity underpinning autoimmunity. Furthermore, the intricate network extends to innate immunity, where nucleotide-binding oligomerization domain-containing protein 2 (*NOD2*) gene variations have been specifically linked to the development of Crohn's disease. Variations in genes such as the *IL-2 receptor* (*IL2R*), IL-23 cytokine receptor (*IL23R*), and *CTLA-4* further underscore the genetic associations with autoimmune diseases, adding layers of complexity to the genetic predispositions involved [37–40]. In some instances, rare autoimmune diseases can be traced back to Mendelian mutations in critical genes such as autoimmune regulator (*AIRE*), *FOXP3*, fas cell surface death receptor (*FAS*), and *CTLA-4*, shedding light on the diverse genetic factors contributing to the intricate tapestry of autoimmune conditions [41].

7.2 Environmental factors

7.2.1 Infections and type I interferons

In the intricate interplay between infections and the immune system, a dual role emerges. On one hand, infections disrupt peripheral T-cell tolerance, setting the stage for autoimmune responses. Notably, viral infections prompt the production of Type I interferons, a key player in the initiation of autoimmune diseases. The phenomenon of molecular mimicry adds another layer, wherein infections generate antigens resembling self-antigens, contributing significantly to the breakdown of immune tolerance [42–45]. Additionally, infections and tissue damage introduce chemical alterations to peripheral tissue antigens, releasing self-antigens. This interaction with autoreactive cells becomes a pivotal factor in the path toward autoimmune diseases, with the cumulative impact of childhood infections potentially serving as the ignition for autoimmunity [46].

7.2.2 Influence of gender, sunlight, and hygiene on autoimmunity

Gender and sunlight exposure, affecting vitamin D_3 levels, have been linked to the prevalence and progression of autoimmune diseases [47]. The "hygiene hypothesis," which posits that exposure to certain infections may protect against autoimmunity, further underscores the impact of environmental factors on autoimmune disease development [48, 49].

8. Autoimmune diseases

8.1 Complexity of autoimmune diseases

Exceeding 130, autoimmune diseases vary in severity, falling into organ-specific and systemic categories [1]. Complexity arises from genetic and phenotypic diversity, with a notable delay in symptom manifestation and diagnostic phenotype development. Autoantibodies aid diagnosis and prognosis, yet the coexistence of multiple disorders complicates management.

8.2 Autoimmune challenges: temporal insights

Understanding autoimmune diseases reveals shared processes with inherent complexities. Challenges include defining early events recognizable only after diagnostic phenotype development. Recent studies on autoantibody development suggest a temporal separation between the onset of an autoimmune response and clinical symptoms.

8.3 Phases of autoimmune disease development

Examining autoimmune disease development unveils four phases: susceptibility, initiation, propagation, and regulation/resolution. The susceptibility phase (Phase I) explores genetic complexities, such as Mendelian patterns in autoimmune polyendocrinopathy-candidiasis-ectodermal dystrophy (APECED) and immune dysregulation, polyendocrinopathy, enteropathy, X-linked (IPEX) syndrome. The initiation phase (Phase II) focuses on adaptive immune responses, emphasizing immunodominance and antigen processing. The propagation phase (Phase III) amplifies the autoimmune process, shedding light on adjuvant properties and innate immune receptors [50].

9. Conclusions

Autoimmune diseases, numbering over a hundred, present significant global health challenges due to their diverse manifestations. The breakdown of immunological tolerance in both central and peripheral mechanisms is crucial for maintaining balance, and disruptions can lead to misguided immune responses. Processes such as negative selection, Treg cell activity, as well as other immune regulatory cells, anergy, and apoptosis are integral to immunological tolerance. Genetic factors, encompassing HLA and non-HLA elements, along with environmental triggers, play pivotal roles in disease initiation. Ongoing research aims to advance diagnosis and treatment, recognizing distinct phases in disease development for potential intervention. Exploring natural regulatory mechanisms provides promising avenues for therapeutic development, acknowledging the active role of target tissues and emphasizing a comprehensive understanding. Future investigations focus on genetic and epigenetic factors, interactions between innate and adaptive immunity, contributions of Treg cells, and the involvement of target tissues in the ongoing amplification process.

Author details

Mourad Aribi
Laboratory of Applied Molecular Biology and Immunology, University of Tlemcen, Tlemcen, Algeria

*Address all correspondence to: mourad.aribi@univ-tlemcen.dz; m_aribi@yahoo.fr; m_aribi@outlook.fr

References

[1] Aribi M. Introductory chapter: Immune system dysfunction and autoimmune diseases. In: Aribi M, editor. Immunopathogenesis Immune-based Therapy for Selected Autoimmune Disorders. London, UK, Rijeka: IntechOpen; 2017. DOI: 10.5772/67671

[2] Dembic Z. Immune system protects integrity of tissues. Molecular Immunology. 2000;**37**:563-569. DOI: 10.1016/s0161-5890(00)00084-5

[3] Dembic Z. Response to Cohn: The immune system rejects the harmful, protects the useful and neglects the rest of microorganisms. Scandinavian Journal of Immunology. 2004;**60**:3-5; discussion 6-8. DOI: 10.1111/j.0300-9475.2004.01451.x

[4] Gol-Ara M, Jadidi-Niaragh F, Sadria R, Azizi G, Mirshafiey A. The role of different subsets of regulatory T cells in immunopathogenesis of rheumatoid arthritis. Arthritis. 2012;**2012**:805875. DOI: 10.1155/2012/805875

[5] Xing Y, Hogquist KA. T-cell tolerance: Central and peripheral. Cold Spring Harbor Perspectives in Biology. 2012;**4**:a006957. DOI: 10.1101/cshperspect.a006957

[6] Greenwood R, Frelinger J. Mechanisms of unresponsiveness: T- and B-cell mediated mechanisms of anergy. Advances in Experimental Medicine and Biology. 2001;**489**:109-117. DOI: 10.1007/978-1-4615-1277-6_10

[7] Gurung P, Kucaba TA, Ferguson TA, Griffith TS. Activation-induced CD154 expression abrogates tolerance induced by apoptotic cells. Journal of immunology Baltimore Md. 2009;**1950**(183):6114-6123. DOI: 10.4049/jimmunol.0901676

[8] Cheru N, Hafler DA, Sumida TS. Regulatory T cells in peripheral tissue tolerance and diseases. Frontiers in Immunology. 2023;**14**:1154575. DOI: 10.3389/fimmu.2023.1154575

[9] Dai J, Fang P, Saredy J, Xi H, Ramon C, Yang W, et al. Metabolism-associated danger signal-induced immune response and reverse immune checkpoint-activated CD40+ monocyte differentiation. Journal of Hematology & Oncology. 2017;**10**:141. DOI: 10.1186/s13045-017-0504-1

[10] Bour-Jordan H, Esensten JH, Martinez-Llordella M, Penaranda C, Stumpf M, Bluestone JA. Intrinsic and extrinsic control of peripheral T-cell tolerance by costimulatory molecules of the CD28/B7 family. Immunological Reviews. 2011;**241**:180-205. DOI: 10.1111/j.1600-065X.2011.01011.x

[11] Crespo J, Sun H, Welling TH, Tian Z, Zou W. T cell anergy, exhaustion, senescence, and stemness in the tumor microenvironment. Current Opinion in Immunology. 2013;**25**:214-221. DOI: 10.1016/j.coi.2012.12.003

[12] Walker LSK. Treg and CTLA-4: Two intertwining pathways to immune tolerance. Journal of Autoimmunity. 2013;**45**:49-57. DOI: 10.1016/j.jaut.2013.06.006

[13] Intlekofer AM, Thompson CB. At the bench: Preclinical rationale for CTLA-4 and PD-1 blockade as cancer immunotherapy. Journal of Leukocyte Biology. 2013;**94**:25-39. DOI: 10.1189/jlb.1212621

[14] Bardhan K, Anagnostou T, Boussiotis VA. The PD1: PD-L1/2 pathway from discovery to clinical

implementation. Frontiers in Immunology. 2016;**7**:550. DOI: 10.3389/fimmu.2016.00550

[15] Murali AK, Mehrotra S. Apoptosis - an Ubiquitous T cell Immunomodulator. Journal of Clinical and Cellular Immunology. 2011;**S3**:2. DOI: 10.4172/2155-9899.S3-002

[16] Hughes P, Bouillet P, Strasser A. Role of Bim and other Bcl-2 family members in autoimmune and degenerative diseases. Current Directions in Autoimmunity. 2006;**9**:74-94. DOI: 10.1159/000090773

[17] van der Vliet HJJ, Nieuwenhuis EE. IPEX as a result of mutations in FOXP3. Clinical & Developmental Immunology. 2007;**2007**:89017. DOI: 10.1155/2007/89017

[18] Aribi M. Immunogenetic aspect of B-cell antigen receptor diversity generation. In: Aribi M, editor. Normal and Malignant B-Cell. London, UK: IntechOpen; 2020. DOI: 10.5772/intechopen.90637

[19] Ferry H, Leung JCH, Lewis G, Nijnik A, Silver K, Lambe T, et al. B-cell tolerance. Transplantation. 2006;**81**:308-315. DOI: 10.1097/01.tp.0000203830.79357.39

[20] Wang Y, Liu J, Burrows PD, Wang J-Y. B cell development and maturation. Advances in Experimental Medicine and Biology. 2020;**1254**:1-22. DOI: 10.1007/978-981-15-3532-1_1

[21] Zoghi S, Masoumi F, Rezaei N. The immune system. In: Clinical Immunology. London, UK: Elsevier; 2023. pp. 1-46. DOI: 10.1016/B978-0-12-818006-8.00005-0

[22] Getahun A. Role of inhibitory signaling in peripheral B cell tolerance. Immunological Reviews. 2022;**307**:27-42. DOI: 10.1111/imr.13070

[23] Abo-Helo N, Vadasz Z, Kessel A, Toubi E. Regulatory B cells. Harefuah. 2016;**155**:50-53, 66

[24] Mauri C, Bosma A. Immune regulatory function of B cells. Annual Review of Immunology. 2012;**30**:221-241. DOI: 10.1146/annurev-immunol-020711-074934

[25] Canny GO, McCormick BA. Bacteria in the intestine, helpful residents or enemies from within? Infection and Immunity. 2008;**76**:3360-3373. DOI: 10.1128/IAI.00187-08

[26] Roncarolo MG, Gregori S, Bacchetta R, Battaglia M, Gagliani N. The biology of T regulatory type 1 cells and their therapeutic application in immune-mediated diseases. Immunity. 2018;**49**:1004-1019. DOI: 10.1016/j.immuni.2018.12.001

[27] Stagg AJ. Intestinal dendritic cells in health and gut inflammation. Frontiers in Immunology. 2018;**9**:2883. DOI: 10.3389/fimmu.2018.02883

[28] Than NG, Hahn S, Rossi SW, Szekeres-Bartho J. Editorial: Fetal-maternal immune interactions in pregnancy. Frontiers in Immunology. 2019;**10**:2729. DOI: 10.3389/fimmu.2019.02729

[29] Huang N, Chi H, Qiao J. Role of regulatory T cells in regulating fetal-maternal immune tolerance in healthy pregnancies and reproductive diseases. Frontiers in Immunology. 2020;**11**:1023. DOI: 10.3389/fimmu.2020.01023

[30] Nevers T, Kalkunte S, Sharma S. Uterine regulatory T cells, IL-10 and hypertension. American Journal of Reproductive Immunology.

2011;**66 Suppl. 1**(Suppl. 1):88-92. DOI: 10.1111/j.1600-0897.2011.01040.x

[31] Jørgensen N, Persson G, Hviid TVF. The Tolerogenic function of regulatory T cells in pregnancy and cancer. Frontiers in Immunology. 2019;**10**:911. DOI: 10.3389/fimmu.2019.00911

[32] Castelli EC, Ramalho J, Porto IOP, Lima THA, Felício LP, Sabbagh A, et al. Insights into HLA-G genetics provided by worldwide haplotype diversity. Frontiers in Immunology. 2014;**5**:476. DOI: 10.3389/fimmu.2014.00476

[33] Ferreira LMR, Meissner TB, Tilburgs T, Strominger JL. HLA-G: At the Interface of maternal-fetal tolerance. Trends in Immunology. 2017;**38**:272-286. DOI: 10.1016/j.it.2017.01.009

[34] Tantengco OAG, Richardson L, Lee A, Kammala A, Silva DMC, Shahin H, et al. Histocompatibility antigen, class I, G (HLA-G)'s role during pregnancy and parturition: A systematic review of the literature. Life Basel Switz. 2021;**11**:1061. DOI: 10.3390/life11101061

[35] Rouas-Freiss N, Paul P, Dausset J, Carosella ED. HLA-G promotes immune tolerance. Journal of Biological Regulators and Homeostatic Agents. 2000;**14**:93-98

[36] Martín-Villa JM, Vaquero-Yuste C, Molina-Alejandre M, Juarez I, Suárez-Trujillo F, López-Nares A, et al. HLA-G: Too much or too little? Role in cancer and autoimmune disease. Frontiers in Immunology. 2022;**13**:796054. DOI: 10.3389/fimmu.2022.796054

[37] Ogura Y, Bonen DK, Inohara N, Nicolae DL, Chen FF, Ramos R, et al. A frameshift mutation in NOD2 associated with susceptibility to Crohn's disease. Nature. 2001;**411**:603-606. DOI: 10.1038/35079114

[38] Chen L, Cao S-Q, Lin Z-M, He S-J, Zuo J-P. NOD-like receptors in autoimmune diseases. Acta Pharmacologica Sinica. 2021;**42**:1742-1756. DOI: 10.1038/s41401-020-00603-2

[39] Harris F, Berdugo YA, Tree T. IL-2-based approaches to Treg enhancement. Clinical and Experimental Immunology. 2023;**211**:149-163. DOI: 10.1093/cei/uxac105

[40] Gaffen SL, Jain R, Garg AV, Cua DJ. The IL-23-IL-17 immune axis: From mechanisms to therapeutic testing. Nature Reviews. Immunology. 2014;**14**:585-600. DOI: 10.1038/nri3707

[41] Abbas AK, Lichtman AH, Pillai S. Basic Immunology: Functions and Disorders of the Immune System. 6th ed. Philadelphia, PA: Elsevier; 2020

[42] Ehl S, Hombach J, Aichele P, Rülicke T, Odermatt B, Hengartner H, et al. Viral and bacterial infections interfere with peripheral tolerance induction and activate CD8+ T cells to cause immunopathology. The Journal of Experimental Medicine. 1998;**187**:763-774. DOI: 10.1084/jem.187.5.763

[43] Enouz S, Carrié L, Merkler D, Bevan MJ, Zehn D. Autoreactive T cells bypass negative selection and respond to self-antigen stimulation during infection. The Journal of Experimental Medicine. 2012;**209**:1769-1779. DOI: 10.1084/jem.20120905

[44] Herbeuval J-P. Editorial: Type 1 interferon in pathologies, autoimmune diseases, and chronic viral infections: Understanding the fascinating biologic role of type 1 interferons. Frontiers in Immunology. 2023;**14**:1239086. DOI: 10.3389/fimmu.2023.1239086

[45] Damian RT. Molecular mimicry: Antigen sharing by parasite and

host and its consequences. The American Naturalist. 1964;**98**:129-149. DOI: 10.2307/2459352

[46] Theofilopoulos AN, Kono DH, Baccala R. The multiple pathways to autoimmunity. Nature Immunology. 2017;**18**:716-724. DOI: 10.1038/ni.3731

[47] Aribi M, Mennechet FJD, Touil-Boukoffa C. Editorial: The role of vitamin D as an immunomodulator. Frontiers in Immunology. 2023;**14**:1186635. DOI: 10.3389/fimmu.2023.1186635

[48] Angum F, Khan T, Kaler J, Siddiqui L, Hussain A. The prevalence of autoimmune disorders in women: A narrative review. Cureus. 2020;**12**:e8094. DOI: 10.7759/cureus.8094

[49] Lahita RG. Sex and gender influence on immunity and autoimmunity. Frontiers in Immunology. 2023;**14**:1142723. DOI: 10.3389/fimmu.2023.1142723

[50] Antiochos B, Rosen A. Mechanisms of autoimmunity. In: Rich RR, Shearer WT, Schroeder H, Frew AJ, editors. Clinical Immunology: Principles and Practice. Amsterdam, Netherlands: Elsevier; 2019. pp. 677-684. DOI: 10.5772/67671

Chapter 2

Intestinal Mucosal Immunity Caused Autoimmune Diseases

Xiaojing Nie, Yuanzhen Zhang, Huanhuan Yang, Yi Chen, Yunfan Zhang, Jingping Cai, Yuxian Tang, Qiuping Fan, Guimei Cai, Ailan Zhao, Yueting Gong and Zihan Dai

Abstract

Autoimmune diseases are a group of chronic inflammatory disorders caused by the imbalance of immune homeostasis and abnormal production of autoantibodies. The etiology of autoimmune diseases involves various factors such as genetic and environmental factors, and the exact pathogenesis remains unclear. The intestinal mucosal immunity including the intestinal epithelial barrier, mucosal immune cells, and innate immune cells cooperatively maintains intestinal immunity against invading pathogens. It has been demonstrated that intestinal mucosal immunity participates in the development of various autoimmune diseases. Dysbiosis of gut microbiota and their metabolite alterations and immune response mediated by intestinal immune cells may be involved in the pathogenesis of systemic lupus erythematosus through multiple mechanisms. When the intestinal mucosal epithelium is damaged, intestinal flora can penetrate the barriers and enter the lamina propria, causing abnormal immune response and inducing the development of Inflammatory Bowel Diseases. Targeting the gut mucosal immune system holds promise for treating autoimmune diseases; therefore, it is necessary to review the role of the gut mucosal immune system in autoimmune diseases and provide guidance for the treatment of autoimmune diseases.

Keywords: intestinal mucosal immunity, autoimmune diseases, gut-associated lymphoid tissue (GALT), gut microbiota, SLE, IBD, type I diabetes

1. Introduction

Autoimmune diseases are characterized by a dysregulated immune response leading to excessive and uncontrolled tissue inflammation. Multiple factors including genetic variation, environmental stimuli, and infection have been implicated as contributing factors to persistent inflammation and pathology. Intestinal mucosal immunity is currently considered to be an important factor in regulating the development of autoimmune diseases. In this chapter, we will discuss the compositions of intestinal mucosal immunity and detail the mechanism of intestinal mucosal immunity involved in the pathogenesis of systemic lupus erythematosus (SLE), inflammatory bowel diseases (IBD), and type 1 diabetes mellitus (T1DM), targeting intestinal mucosal immunity for providing new treatment for autoimmune diseases.

2. Summarize

2.1 History of the development of intestinal mucosal immunity

In ancient China, there was a technique to prevent smallpox by grinding the pox scabs of smallpox patients into powder and blowing it into the nasal cavity of healthy people to prevent them from contracting the smallpox virus. This form of immunity was based on protective immunity to the nasal mucosa. With the development of microbiology, Alexandre Besredka [1] developed a method to obtain immune protection by oral administration of bacteria, also known as oral vaccine. This approach also mediated a protective immune response through the mucosa of the digestive tract. With the development of various vaccines, mucosal immunology was gradually developed. These included the discovery of Peyer's patches at the end of the ileum in the late 17th century [2], the discovery of mucosal tolerance mechanisms in the gut, the identification of secretory and serotype IgA, and the discovery of M cells in the gut in 1982, among others.

2.2 Physiopathology of intestinal mucosal immunity

With the development of various vaccines and modern immunology, intestinal mucosal immunology has been greatly promoted, and mucosal immunity is closely related to both disease and physiology. In terms of pathological regulation, many pathogens including bacteria and viruses infect the body through the mucosal system [3]. Mucosal immunity is also closely related to inflammation and tumors. In addition, mucosal immunity has a very important role in physiological regulation. It is able to interact with commensal bacteria and can mediate the regulation of immunity and neurology, immunity, and metabolism.

2.3 Research methods of intestinal mucosal immunity

The study of intestinal mucosal immunity can be performed using various research methods such as histology and immunohistochemistry [3], which provide information on the distribution and activation status of immune cells within the intestinal mucosa as well as on the expression levels of cytokines and chemokines. Animal models such as germ-free mice, as an effective tool for gut flora research, are in a state of absolute sterility from the embryonic stage, allowing better elucidation of the mechanisms driving gut microbes in many diseases [4]. Combining transcriptomic and microbiomic studies can explore the relationship with host phenotype from the perspectives of host genes and flora, respectively, and can also reveal that key microorganisms regulate host gene expression through correlation analysis [5]. Proteomics enables direct study of protein molecular differences in immune cells between samples, revealing new diagnostic markers and therapeutic targets related to immune disorders [6]. In addition to these approaches, recent advances in single-cell sequencing allow a more detailed understanding of the heterogeneity of the immune cell population within the intestinal mucosa [7]. A large number of in vitro culture and molecular biology techniques are now available for human microbiome studies, which can be used to detect and analyze microbial community composition, species diversity, and effects on human cellular pathways. With the rapid development of modern biomolecular science, we determined the gut microbiota using high-throughput sequencing technology based mainly on 16SrRNA/18SrRNA genes. Through bioinformatics principles and statistical analysis of a large amount of data, we can analyze the diversity of intestinal microorganisms and obtain the type and distribution of intestinal flora to make scientific judgments on the health status of the body through such dynamic changes. In addition, through microbial rRNA gene sequencing, macrogenomics, macrotranscriptomics, and nontargeted metabolomics combined with the core strategy of "whole microbiome association analysis (MWAS)", we can accurately decode the composition, function, and expression profiles of the flora and uncover key biomarkers to elucidate [8].

In summary, the study of intestinal mucosal immunity is complex and requires the use of multiple research approaches; by combining these approaches, researchers can gain insight into the complex interactions between immune cells and intestinal microbiota in regulating intestinal mucosal immunity and the impact of various interventions on this process.

3. Compositions of intestinal mucosal immunity

The components of intestinal mucosal immunity include gut-associated lymphoid tissue (GALT), the intestinal mucosal epithelium, and gut microbiota (see **Figure 1**).

3.1 Gut-associated lymphoid tissue

GALT composed of Peyer's patches (PPS), laminar propria lymphocytes, and intraepithelial lymphocytes is an important component of intestinal acquired

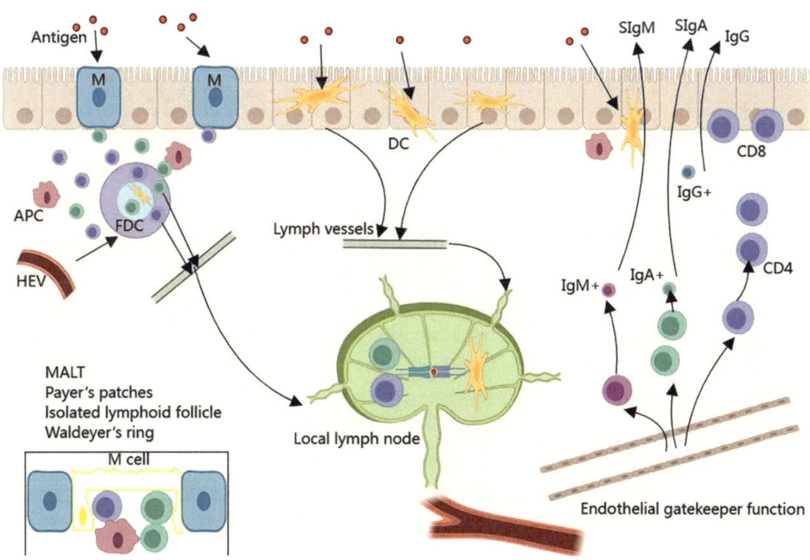

Figure 1.
Compositions of intestinal mucosal immunity.

immunity [9]. As the largest lymphoid tissue in the body, GALT recognizes exogenous and abnormal antigens in a timely manner by uptake, processing, and presentation of antigens. After specific recognition of foreign antigens, GALT promotes the production of cytokines and antibodies to coordinate the immune response. In addition, it activates T lymphocytes and B lymphocytes to establish an effective adaptive immune response and induce a mucosal immune response or immune tolerance [9].

Peyer junction was mainly distributed in the intestinal wall and the inferior mucosa on the opposite side of the attachment margin of the mesentery, which is essential for the induction and initiation of mucosal immunity. In the lamina propria of the mucosa of the GI, there is diffuse lymphoid tissue made of lymphocytes and dendritic cells (DCs). Within the lamina propria, macrophages, mature plasma cells, and sporadic T lymphocytes and B lymphocytes can be found. The role of these cells is to capture and process antigens, which secondly reach regional lymph nodes and start the immune response, eventually followed by the production of immunoglobulin (Ig)A, IgG, and IgM. The myeloid compartment represented by macrophages and DCs is crucial for the maintenance of intestinal tolerance and the activation of T-cell immunity [10, 11]. Intraepithelial lymphocytes (IELs) of the lamina propria are heterogeneous and are represented by a mixed population of T-lymphocytes: mainly differentiation (CD)4(+) cells and some CD8(+) ones. Intraepithelial lymphocytes are a group of smaller lymphocytes distributed among intestinal epithelial cells, mostly located in the columnar epithelium of the intestine and mainly include TCRαβ+ CD8αα + T-cells, TCRγδ+ CD8αα + T-cells, TCRαβ+ CD4+ T-cells and TCRαβ+ CD8αβ + T-cells [12]. They comprise the vast majority of intestinal epithelial cells (IECs) in the small intestine and are essential in maintaining immune homeostasis in the intestinal territory such as keeping the integrity of the gut barrier [13].

3.2 The intestinal mucosal epithelium

The intestinal mucosal epithelium constitutes the physical and chemical barrier of the intestinal mucosal immune system including the epithelial layer and the mucus layer on the surface of epithelial cells [14]. The epithelial layer consists of a single layer of closely connected IECs, composed of a number of cell types such as goblet cells, absorptive enterocytes, enteroendocrine cells, Paneth cells, microfold (M) cells, and tuft cells [14]. IECs separate the internal and external environment of the body and can resist the antigens, toxins, pathogens, and microorganisms in the intestinal lumen. However, IEC also plays an important role in absorbing nutrients present in the intestinal lumen [15]. The mucus layer is the first line of defense in the intestinal mucosal epithelium. Paneth cells are capable of secreting antimicrobial peptides (AMPs) to defend against external pathogens or intestinal bacteria. The mucus layer and AMPs constitute the mucosal barrier to prevent the invasion of symbiotic bacteria.

Additionally, there were scattered intraepithelial lymphocytes (IELs) between closely connected IECs [16]. Approximately 90% of all IEL express T-cell receptors (TCR) [17]. In the small intestine, approximately 1 IEL per 10 IEC [18]. According to different expression profiles of T-cell receptors (TCRs), the TCR+ IELs can be divided into the following two groups: TCRαβ and TCRγδ [12]. Based on the large quantities and special locations, the IELs play an important role in maintaining intestinal immune tolerance and regulating intestinal immunity.

3.3 Gut microbiota

Gut microbiota is a system of microorganisms that resides in the host gut and lives in symbiosis with the host, including bacteria, fungi, and viruses [19]. The gut microbiota and its metabolites maintain the integrity of the intestinal mucosal barrier and participate in the maintenance of the body's mucosal immune system by regulating innate and adaptive immunity.

Intestinal commensal bacteria promote the development and functional maturation of the host intestinal mucosal immune system. Work in germ-free (GF) mice showed that GF animals have a myriad of intestinal immune defects, including impaired development of GALTs fewer intestinal IgA-secreting plasma cells, smaller PPs, fewer IELs, Treg and Th17 cells [20–23]. However, most of these deficiencies can be corrected by recolonization with a health-associated mouse commensal microbiota [24, 25]. In normal conditions, intestinal epithelial cells act as a barrier to keep immune cells residing in the intestinal mucosa separate from intestinal microorganisms, thus building a microbial-host symbiosis. In turn, gut microbiota maintains the integrity of the intestinal mechanical barrier. Studies have shown that bacterial metabolites play an important role in maintaining intestinal integrity. Short-chain fatty acids (SCFAs) promote the proliferation of intestinal epithelial cells and promote mucin secretion by goblet cells, which protects the intestinal epithelium from damage by acid and intestinal lumen contents [26]. Furthermore, in vitro experiments have also demonstrated that butyrate can upregulate MUC2 expression by activating the MUC2 promoter and altering histone modifications in this region [27]. Additionally, bacteria components such as lipopolysaccharide (LPS) and flagellin can be recognized by pattern recognition receptors IECs, which promote cell proliferation and the production of cytokines, antimicrobial peptides, and mucus [28].

Microbiota plays another important role in the intestinal mucosal immune system, that is, the intestinal commensal bacteria involved in immune response and immune modulation. Many studies have shown that dysbiosis of microbiota increases host susceptibility to a variety of immune, inflammatory, and allergic diseases, which may be because of the gut microbiota involved in CD4+ T-cell differentiation via different pathways as well as in the induction of sIgA [29–31]. Specifically, it can be divided into the following points: 1) Microbiota can affect Th17 differentiation and participate in the mucosal immune system defense against pathogens. For example, after SFB is colonized, naive CD4 T-cells migrate olites can induce the differentiation of Treg cells, participate in the immune reg to the small intestine and differentiate into IL-17A-producing Th17 cells, whose products stimulate the production of antimicrobial peptides by IECs [32]. 2) Microbiota and its metabulation and maintenance of immune homeostasis together with Th17 cells [31]. 3) Microbiota can regulate the intestinal T follicular helper cells, which can participate in the production of high-affinity antibodies by B-cells and it is thought to be the chief cell regulating B-cells in germinal centers. As the SFB colonized in IL-21R-deficient mice, the number of IgA plasmablasts and plasma cells decreased significantly [33]. 4) Microbiota can affect the accumulation of sIgA-producing plasma cells and also affect the diversity of IgA in the lymphocyte tissues of the gut [34].

Therefore, the interaction between the microbiota and the intestinal immune system is essential to maintain intramucosal homeostasis. However, ecological dysbiosis can lead to intestinal diseases when the balanced intestinal microbial community is altered.

4. Intestinal mucosal immunity and autoimmune diseases

There is a close yet complex link between intestinal flora and immune-related diseases. Dysbiosis of intestinal flora plays an important role in the development of immune-related diseases including SLE, IBD, and T1DM (**Figure 2**).

4.1 Systemic lupus erythematosus

SLE is an autoimmune disease characterized by the presence of nuclear autoantibodies and complex immune inflammation involving multiple organs. The pathogenesis is not fully understood. Some factors such as molecular genetics, epigenetics, immunomodulation, ethnicity, possible environmental influences (ultraviolet light, drugs, and infection) and sex hormones are associated with its occurrence [35]. Gut microbiota and their metabolites have been proposed to be involved in SLE development and progression through intestinal mucosal immunity [36].

Increasing evidence supports that dysbiosis of gut microbiota is associated with lupus pathogenesis. The number of non-pathogenic bacteria such as Bifidobacterium and Bacteroides fragilis in the intestine of SLE patients was significantly reduced compared with normal controls, whereas the number of conditionally pathogenic bacteria such as Ruminococcus gnavus and Enterococcus gallinarum was significantly increased compared with the normal group [36]. It has been indicated that gut microbiota metabolites such as SCFAs amino acids and lipids are correlated with SLE. Most of the SCFA that exist in the gut are acetate, propionate, and butyrate [37]. The immunoregulatory functions of SCFA range from anti-inflammatory, T cell, and

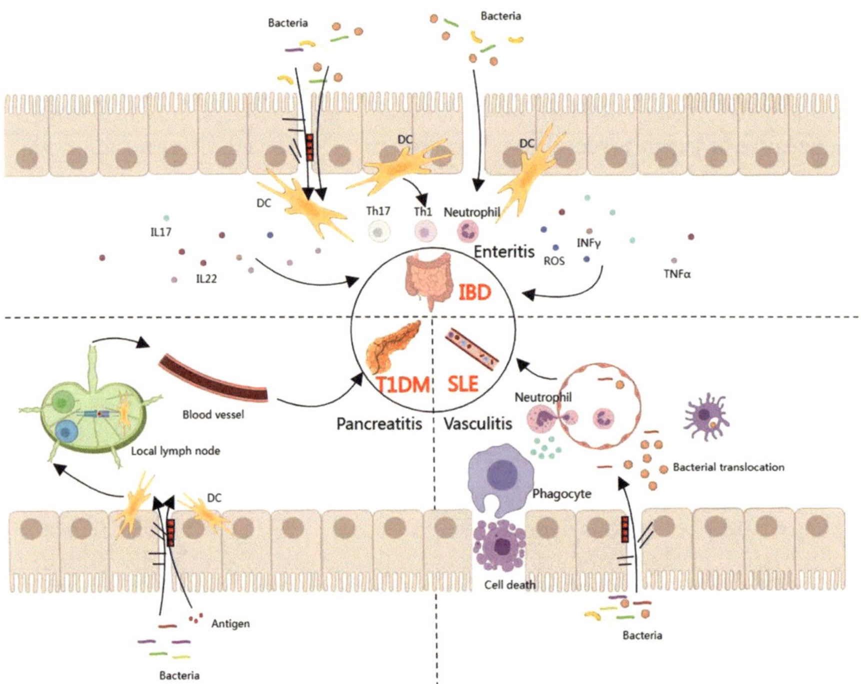

Figure 2.
Association between intestinal mucosal immunity and immunologic diseases.

epigenetic pathways. Bacteroides and Negativicutes produce propionate through the succinate pathway. However, butyrate was mainly produced by phylum Firmicutes via the acetate CoA-transferase pathway [38]. Butyrate decreases permeability by accelerating the assembly of tight junctions via the activation AMPK [39]. Bifidobacterium species increase gut barrier integrity by producing acetate, which increases the expression of the tight junction gene occludin [40]. Because most butyrate-producing bacteria belong to the Firmicutes phylum, inflammation and impaired gut barrier integrity may be induced by the decreased relative abundance of Firmicutes in SLE patients [36]. Changes in intestinal flora associated with changes in lupus disease, such as the abundance of Streptococcus, Campylobacter, Veillonella, Clostridiacae, and Lachnospiraceae, were positively correlated with SLE disease activity. The abundance of Bifidobacterium was negatively correlated with lupus activity. In addition [41], the intestinal flora of SLE patients with lupus nephritis and gastrointestinal damage showed a decrease in the thick-walled phylum, an increase in the Aspergillus phylum, and a relative increase in the Aspergillus phylum, Enterobacteriaceae, and Shigella coli.

Gut microbiota influences SLE through different mechanisms. First, the abnormal gut microbiota translocation results in what is known as the "leaky gut," triggering the systemic autoimmune response [36]. The imbalance of gut microbiota can compromise intestinal permeability, allowing the passage of antigens and bacteria in the lumen to the blood circulation, which causes leaky gut syndromes that exacerbate lupus immunopathogenesis [42]. It has been reported that toll-like receptors (TLRs) contribute to lupus pathogenesis by sensing harmful bacteria coming from gut microbiota through microbial translocation, especially in the presence of a leaky gut. Activation of TLR4 with LPS inducing the release of CD14 from monocytes contributes to the pathogenesis of SLE and exacerbates its development [43]. Second, interference with immune cells in the lamina propria leads to the development of SLE. Aberrant monocyte/macrophage surface markers were expressed in cells from SLE patients, including Fcγ receptors, ICAM-1 (intercellular adhesion molecule-1, CD54), CD40, MHC II, type-1 interferon-stimulated genes, and sialoadhesin (Siglec-1,CD169) [44]. Besides the deregulations of monocyte/macrophage surface markers, macrophages in SLE patients also have a defect in phagocytosis. Ineffective clearance of dying cells and debris by macrophages may provide a source of autoantigens for the development of autoantibodies in SLE disease [45]. TLRs are a type of cell transmembrane signal transduction protein in the innate immune system, which recognizes microbial-related molecular patterns to trigger different immune responses. MYD88 is the main linker molecule of the TLR signal transduction pathway. Most studies suggest that the TLR/MYD88 signaling pathway plays an important role in restricting the penetration of the intestinal microbiome and preventing mucosal immune regulation disorders, and it is essential for maintaining a normal intestinal mucosal barrier and regulating intestinal homeostasis [46]. LPS mostly coming from the intestinal lumen is recognized by TLR4 and the interaction between them has been proven to promote the inflammatory response and exacerbate the development of SLE [47]. Studies found that the high level of plasma LPS in patients with SLE caused by the impaired intestinal mucosal barrier was positively correlated with the level of serum anti-double-stranded DNA antibodies, which suggested that the increased intestinal permeability was beneficial to LPS in order to penetrate the intestinal epithelium and translocate into the tissue to promote the progression of disease [48]. Moreover, altered inflammatory cytokine production from monocytes/macrophages has also been found in SLE patients. Elevated monocyte counts, increased CD16 expression, and IL-6 production in monocytes were found in SLE patients. Plasma sCD14 and IL-6 cytokines released by monocytes in response to LPS are increased in lupus patients relative to controls [49]. Macrophage-mediated maintenance of tolerance and prevention of proinflammatory responses to TLR ligands at the intestinal mucosal site is important for mucosal immunity. Altered TLR-mediated innate immune responses in intestinal macrophages may play a key role in SLE disease pathogenesis [50]. Finally, The cross-reactivity between certain bacteria antigens with specific autoantibodies has been recognized as the main factor of leaky gut syndrome in lupus. Autoantibodies to the 60 kDa Ro protein are common in SLE patients. It was found early that the lupus autoantigen Ro60 cross-reacted with the Ebstein-Barr virus nuclear antigen-1 (EBNA-1), suggesting that lupus humoral autoimmunity was initiated via molecular mimicry of EBNA-1 and Ro60 antigens [51]. Colonization of Bacteroides thetaiotaomicron in lupus mice was found to enhance the expression of Ro60 antigen followed by deposition of immune complex causing lupus nephritis [41]. Gut microbiota maintains a symbiotic relationship with the host. It uses the energy and sources of the host to ensure its growth and releases metabolites, which in turn influence the host's metabolism.

Impaired composition and function of gut microbiota have been associated with several autoimmune diseases including SLE. These mechanisms include leaky gastrointestinal tract disturbing its equilibrium, crossreactivity of microbial proteins with self-antigens, and dysregulation of both innate and adaptive immunity. These alterations lead to self-tolerance breakdown and autoantibodies production. Therefore, it is important to decipher the commensal bacteria profiles associated with SLE because these may guide the scientific community to a better understanding of the disease.

4.2 Inflammatory bowel diseases

IBD, which mainly includes Crohn's disease (CD) and ulcerative colitis (UC), are chronic, nonspecific, relapsing, and inflammatory disease mainly involving the gastrointestinal tract [52]. The global burden of IBD remains a persistent health problem. The prevalence of IBD in Europe, North America, and other Western countries exceeds 0.3% and is increasing in many newly industrialized countries [53, 54]. The etiology of IBD is not yet fully understood, and it has been proven to be related to complex factors such as genetics, environment, intestinal microbes, and immunity [55].

In recent years, studies have suggested that intestinal mucosal immunity plays a pivotal role. Several clinical studies have shown that UC and CD patients have different degrees of intestinal flora dysbiosis with reduced intestinal flora diversity, reduced intestinal probiotics, and increased pathogenic bacteria [56]. Sequencing of intestinal flora revealed that probiotics such as Bifidobacterium and Lactobacillus were significantly reduced and pathogenic bacteria such as Enterococcus and Enterobacteriaceae were increased in the intestinal flora of UC patients compared with healthy adults, whereas probiotics such as Lactobacillus, Bacteroides, and Rumenococcus were reduced and Actinobacillus, Aspergillus, and Enterobacteriaceae were increased in CD patients. It was found that the site of lesion, disease activity, and duration of disease in IBD patients have an effect on their intestinal flora. Besides, the disease activity of IBD patients also had an effect on the intestinal flora with an increase in disease activity index in CD patients associated with an increase in Enterobacteriaceae, but no association was found between disease activity index and intestinal flora in UC patients [57]. Patients with IBD not only have dysregulated numbers and types of intestinal flora but also abnormalities in the function of intestinal flora [58]. A study in a mouse model of colitis found that butyrate, one of the SCFA, maintains Th17/Treg balance in the gut and exerts anti-inflammatory effects [59]. Certain intestinal bacteria such as F. saccharivorans may also exert their anti-inflammatory effects by producing SCFA, whereas butyrate-producing flora such as Roseburia hominis (R. hominis) and E. pumilus are reduced in patients with UC and their reduction may have contributed to the overexpression of proinflammatory factors in human intestinal cells, which can cause inflammation [60]. In addition, smoking exacerbates the symptoms of enteritis in CD patients [61]. External factors such as smoking, diet, medications, and emotions act on the intestinal flora, causing a decrease in the abundance of SCFAs-producing organisms (e.g., B. thicketi) and an increase in the abundance of pathogenic organisms (e.g., Aspergillus, Bacteroidetes), which can contribute to the development of intestinal inflammation in susceptible individuals [55].

The pathogenesis of IBD has not been fully elucidated, and a large number of studies have found that the intestinal flora plays an important role and that intestinal mucosal immune disorders may be the initiating factor in the pathogenesis of IBD. Barrier disruption of the intestinal mucosal epithelium is an important pathogenetic feature of IBD. When the epithelium is damaged, the mechanical barrier permeability is greatly increased, and intestinal lumen such as macromolecular proteins and pathogenic bacteria can enter the lamina propria through the broken mechanical barrier, inducing the development of IBD [62]. With the gradual development of high-throughput assays, IncRNA, as a new molecule in biology, has been shown to activate intestinal inflammatory genes, damage epithelial cells, and disrupt intercellular tight junctions leading to an abnormal increase in the permeability of the mechanical barrier of the intestinal mucosa and affecting the intestinal barrier, which is an important precursor alteration in the pathogenesis of IBD [63]. When IBD occurs, the mucus barrier function is absent. It has been shown that in patients with active UC and animal models, intestinal mucus granules are reduced and mucus is thinned, allowing microorganisms to be exposed to the surface of intestinal mucosal epithelial cells [63]; whereas in patients with CD, the production of mucus is instead increased, which is considered to be a result of the disruption of the integrity of the mucus network by the production of sulfides by a number of specific bacteria in the intestinal mucus, which in turn increases the host's contact with microorganisms and toxins, and induces inflammatory responses [64]. Changes in the intestinal microbiota are accompanied by the thinning of the intestinal mucus layer leading to barrier rupture, epithelial defects, and displacement of intestinal flora across the barrier to induce DC and macrophage activation, which induces inflammatory CD4T cell infiltration into intestinal tissues [65]. Normal intestinal immunity protects against pathogen invasion but a sustained, abnormal immune response can damage the intestinal wall [66]. Patients with IBD have been found to have abnormalities in both innate and adaptive immunity, with differences in the immunologic profile of UC and CD. Patients with IBD have increased levels of pro-inflammatory Th1 and Th17 cells. This infiltration is accompanied by an increase in the number of Th2 cells and a deficit in the number of immunosuppressive cells (e.g., Tregs) [67] . Inflammatory T cells direct the function of cells with innate immunity such as epithelial cells, fibroblasts, and phagocytes, thus stimulating a sustained hyperreactivity to microbial antigens and causing tissue damage and chronic intestinal inflammation [68]. Therefore, when the physical, chemical, and mucus barriers are compromised, intestinal flora can penetrate the barriers and enter the lamina propria, inducing an abnormal immune response.

Because of the adverse effects and ineffectiveness of some of the standardized therapies for IBD, the search for new and effective therapies has always been a goal pursued by researchers and clinicians. Currently, researchers are committed to treating IBD by restoring gut microbial homeostasis and improving intestinal inflammation through the use of probiotics, prebiotics, synbiotics, and fecal microbial transplants as complementary and alternative medications, among others. Fecal microbial transplantation is the process of transplanting functional flora from the feces of a healthy population into the gastrointestinal tract of a patient. The use of FMT in IBD patients is expected to treat the disease by restoring gut microbial homeostasis in patients. Currently, four clinical randomized controlled studies of FMT for the treatment of UC have been reported, three of which concluded that FMT was effective in inducing remission of UC [69–71]. A recent network meta-analysis in UC has described that when compared with available targeted pharmacotherapies, fecal microbiota transplantation (FMT) has a comparable effect in inducing clinical remission, clinical response, and endoscopic remission [72]. Data from the US clinicaltrial.gov website show that several RCTs of FMT for CD are underway but no relevant RCTs have been reported. One recent systematic review of FMT for IBD, which counted the results of 11 studies in CD, showed a 50.5% remission rate of FMT in CD (42/83) [73]. In a meta-analysis of 12 studies, FMT was associated with clinical remission and clinical response in 62% and 79% of patients with CD, respectively [74]. This shows that FMT has some potential for the treatment of IBD and it may provide a new therapeutic pathway for patients with IBD, especially for those who have failed to be treated with traditional methods but more clinical studies need to be conducted to confirm this.

4.3 Type I diabetes mellitus

Type 1 diabetes mellitus (T1DM), also known as insulin-dependent diabetes mellitus, usually starts in adolescence. T1DM patients have absolute insulin deficiency due to autoimmune destruction of pancreatic beta cells so exogenous insulin is needed to control blood glucose [75]. In recent years, due to rapid economic development and unhealthy lifestyle, type I diabetes has become a metabolic disease that seriously threatens human life expectancy.

Because of the many factors involved in the pathogenesis and the close relationship between them, the etiology of the disease is still not fully understood. Recent studies have found that the intestinal microbial diversity and abundance are lower in TDM patients than in healthy controls, with lower abundance of both the Actinobacteria and thick-walled bacteria phylum, lower abundance of Lactobacillus, Bifidobacterium, Clostridium/Proctobacteria and Prevotella, and higher abundance of the Mycobacterium phylum [76]. Follow-up studies also found that in quantitative experiments of intestinal metabolites, the metabolic production of intestinal butyrate was significantly different in normal healthy individuals compared with type 1 diabetics, and levels of butyrate-producing bacteria were significantly lower in type I diabetics compared with normal healthy individuals based on quantitative comparisons of intestinal flora [77].

The intestinal microbiota may act by influencing intestinal permeability, molecular mimicry, and modulation of the innate and adaptive immune systems. Studies have shown that when the intestinal barrier is compromised, pancreatic-draining lymph node T cells, particularly diabetic-derived CD8+ T cells, will be activated and will proliferate, promoting insulitis [77]. In addition, many other studies have shown that changes in certain microorganisms such as Clostridium perfringens, invisible Dialister, Gemella sanguinis, and Bifidobacterium longum are associated with impaired intestinal integrity and increased risk of T1DM [78]. When intestinal permeability is increased, intestinal toxins, food antigens, and infection factors can transit from the gastrointestinal lumen to the intestinal mucosal components and eventually to the pancreatic lymph nodes, inducing or exacerbating TID. A recent proteomic analysis also showed that the intestinal flora associated with host proteins related to the maintenance of mucus barrier function and microvillus adhesion is depleted in patients with new-onset T1DM [79]. In addition, children at high risk for T1DM have increased intestinal permeability and are associated with altered intestinal flora [80]. Therefore, the intestinal flora and its metabolites may be able to influence the development of T1DM by altering the barrier function of the intestine. Microbial peptide mimics produced by Clostridium perfringens to mimic sequences in the insulin b chain and trigger or participate in the immune response to T1DM development. Flavobacterium, Bacillus cereus, and Enterobacter mori LMG 25706 (Leptotrichia goodfellowii, Flavobacteriia bacterium, Bacillus cereus, and Enterobacter mori LMG 25706) also possess diabetic IGRP206–214 homologous peptide that can induce or accelerate T1DM through molecular mimicry [81]. The interaction between gut microbes and immunity is also crucial in the development and pathogenesis of T1DM. For example, studies in animals lacking myeloid differentiation primary response protein 88 (MyD88) have highlighted the link between gut flora-induced alterations in innate immunity and the risk of T1DM. MyD88 induces toll-like receptors in the intestinal flora, triggers different toll-like receptors, and induces pre- and anti-diabetic signals to promote cellular responses to LPS [75, 82]. A study by Gülden et al. revealed novel innate immune pathways influenced by gut flora in T1DM development. They found that knockdown of the β-interferon TIR structural region articulation protein (TIR-domain-containing adaptor inducing interferon-β, TRIF), another key articulator protein downstream of the TLR, protected NOD mice from diabetes. Importantly, different gut flora characteristics were found in TRIF-deficient NOD mice compared with wild-type NOD mice, suggesting that the protective effect of TRIF deficiency is mediated by altered gut flora [83]. Some specific intestinal bacteria have the ability to regulate T cell subsets and functions. Listeria monocytogenes can induce Th1 responses, whereas segmented filamentous bacteria can enhance Th17 responses. Altered schedule flora and Clostridium perfringens consortia have the ability to induce regulatory T cells [64, 84]. In addition, altered intestinal flora can increase the number of type 1 regulatory T (Tr1) cells in the intestine [85]. These Tr1 cells can migrate to the periphery, inhibit the activation of effector T cells, and reduce the incidence of diabetes.

In addition, the gut microbiome also plays a key role in the development of certain subpopulations of innate T-cells such as mucosal associated invariant T (MAIT) cells. Mucosal associated invariant T (MAIT) cells are innate T-like cells that recognize derivatives of bacterial riboflavin metabolites presented by MHC-Ib associated protein 1 (MR1) molecules and are important effector cells in mucosal immunity [86]. Upon activation, MAIT cells produce several proinflammatory cytokines such as IFN-γ and IL-17A and exhibit cytotoxic effects on cells infected with certain pathogens [87]. In recent years, changes in circulating MAIT compartments such as T1DM have been observed in a variety of autoimmune diseases. In the intestinal mucosa, MAIT cells may play a protective role by producing IL-17A and IL-22, two key cytokines in intestinal homeostasis [88–91]. This increased pathogenic response is associated with loss of intestinal integrity, decreased expression of tight junction proteins, and abnormal mucus distribution. Thus, the gut microbiota may be a key regulator of T1DM pathogenesis.

5. Treatment progress of autoimmune diseases based on intestinal mucosal immunity

Traditional treatment methods have played a significant role in controlling and managing autoimmune diseases primarily including glucocorticoids, immunosuppressants, and intravenous immunoglobulins. With in-depth research on the mucosal immune system and autoimmune diseases, emerging treatment approaches are continually emerging, providing new options for improving treatment outcomes and reducing side effects.

Interventions targeting key regulatory molecules of mucosal immune responses and suppressing or enhancing specific immune pathways or signaling molecules can precisely modulate the activity of the immune system [92]. In mucosal immune responses, prominent proinflammatory cytokines and growth factors include IL-1β, interferon-gamma, TNF-alpha (TNF-α), and IL-6. Anifrolumab targets and inhibits signaling through the type I interferon receptor subunit 1 and has shown efficacy in SLE evidenced by improvements in various clinical outcomes including mucocutaneous and musculoskeletal manifestations, lower flare rates, relapse rates, and successful tapering from glucocorticoids to ≤7.5 mg/day [93]. Anti-tumor necrosis TNF-α antibody drugs such as infliximab, adalimumab, and certolizumab pegol have demonstrated significant clinical success and are widely used as first-line therapy for IBD [42].

Enhancement or modulation of mucosal immune responses can be achieved by introducing modified immune cells into the patient's body. The most commonly used approach currently is the fusion of T cells with antigen-specific chimeric molecules known as chimeric antigen receptor T-cell (CAR-T) therapy. In 2021, Dimitrios M et al. reported the data on the use of anti-CD19 CAR-T cells in patients with refractory SLE, showing rapid clinical remission and no significant adverse reactions accompanied by sustained depletion of circulating B lymphocytes and rapid disappearance of serum anti-DNA antibodies [94]. Toxicities associated with this therapy mainly include cytokine release syndrome, which can be life-threatening; but in most cases, effective specific strategies including the use of monoclonal antibodies blocking IL-6 activity can be employed to mitigate the release of proinflammatory cytokines. CAR-T cell therapy represents an interesting and promising approach for SLE treatment but further randomized controlled trials are needed to evaluate its efficacy.

The structure and function of the gut microbiome can influence the balance of the mucosal immune system. Microbiota-based therapies include fecal microbiota transplantation, probiotics, prebiotics, and postbiotics, with the basic principle of introducing or promoting potentially beneficial microorganisms in patients. They have been extensively studied in diseases such as IBD and type 1 diabetes [76]. For example, Butzner JD et al. found that butyrate enemas effectively treated ulcerative colitis and UC patients, whereas Sun J et al. discovered that injection of butyrate into spontaneously diabetic NOD mice controlled pancreatic inflammation by regulating cathelicidin-related antimicrobial peptide production, thereby suppressing the development of autoimmune diabetes [95]. Although microbiota-based therapies are still in the early stages, ongoing research and clinical trials suggest that this approach may be the most effective method for developing IBD treatments.

The relationship between the mucosal immune system and autoimmune diseases is complex and diverse. In-depth understanding of abnormalities in the mucosal immune system and their interaction with specific diseases is of significant importance in developing novel therapeutic approaches for these diseases. Further research on the association between the mucosal immune system and autoimmune diseases contributes to a better understanding of the underlying mechanisms and provides new insights and strategies for treatment and prevention.

6. Conclusion

The role of intestinal mucosal immunity in autoimmune diseases has received increasing attention. Reduced diversity and abnormal strain distribution of intestinal flora have been detected in patients with a variety of autoimmune diseases, and the possible mechanisms involved in immune disorders include: translocation and molecular mimicry of the flora, dysregulation of flora, SCFAs inducing immune imbalance, epitope expansion, and bystander activation. The relevance of intestinal mucosal immunity to autoimmune diseases was further investigated by combining a preclinical model (a germ-free mouse model) and host multi-omics characterization approaches (e.g., 16SrRNA/18SrRNA genes, high-throughput sequencing, macrogenomics, macrotranscriptomics and nontargeted metabolomics, transcriptomics). This provides a possibility to develop interventions based on intestinal flora for the treatment of autoimmune diseases.

Acknowledgements

This work was supported in part by the National Natural Science Foundation of China (project no. 81300583), Science and Technology Innovation Project of Fujian Province (project no. 2019Y9043), Key Project of Social Development of Fujian Province of China (project no. 2019Y0069), Key Project of Social Development of Fujian Province of China (project no. 2023Y0068) and Foundation of The 900th Hospital of Joint Logistic Team (project no. 2021MS15, 2021JQ10, 2022MS30, 2022ZD05, 2023ON02).

Conflict of interest

The authors declare no conflict of interest.

Author details

Xiaojing Nie[1,2,3*], Yuanzhen Zhang[1,2,3†], Huanhuan Yang[1,2†], Yi Chen[1,2,3], Yunfan Zhang[1], Jingping Cai[3], Yuxian Tang[1], Qiuping Fan[1], Guimei Cai[3], Ailan Zhao[1], Yueting Gong[3] and Zihan Dai[1]

1 Fuzong Clinical Medical College of Fujian Medical University, Fuzhou, China

2 Department of Pediatrics, The 900th Hospital of Joint Logistic Support Force, Fuzhou, China

3 Department of Pediatrics, Affiliated Dongfang Hospital, Xiamen University, Fuzhou, China

*Address all correspondence to: searchnj051@126.com

† These authors contributed equally.

References

[1] Rietschel ET, Cavaillon JM. Richard Pfeiffer and Alexandre Besredka: Creators of the concept of endotoxin and anti-endotoxin. Microbes and Infection. 2003;**5**(15):1407-1414. DOI: 10.1016/j.micinf.2003.10.003

[2] CDC. Update: Mass vaccination with oral poliovirus vaccine--Asia and Europe, 1996. MMWR. Morbidity and Mortality Weekly Report. 1996;**45**(42):911-914

[3] Perez-Lopez A, Behnsen J, Nuccio SP, et al. Mucosal immunity to pathogenic intestinal bacteria. Nature Reviews. Immunology. 2016;**16**(3):135-148. DOI: 10.1038/nri.2015.17

[4] Bamias G, Arseneau KO, Cominelli F. Mouse models of inflammatory bowel disease for investigating mucosal immunity in the intestine. Current Opinion in Gastroenterology. 2017;**33**(6):411-416. DOI: 10.1097/MOG.0000000000000402

[5] James KR, Elmentaite R, Teichmann SA, et al. Redefining intestinal immunity with single-cell transcriptomics. Mucosal Immunology. 2022;**15**(4):531-541. DOI: 10.1038/s41385-021-00470-y

[6] Wen J, Niu X, Chen S, et al. Chitosan oligosaccharide improves the mucosal immunity of small intestine through activating SIgA production in mice: Proteomic analysis. International Immunopharmacology. 2022;**109**:108826. DOI: 10.1016/j.intimp.2022.108826

[7] Lemme-Dumit JM. mSphere of influence: Organoids and single-cell sequencing, a powerful combination to uncover epithelial and immune cell interactions in the human gut environment. mSphere. 2020;**5**(4):e00722-20. DOI: 10.1128/mSphere.00722-20

[8] Kanangat S, Skaljic I. Microbiome analysis, the immune response and transplantation in the era of next generation sequencing. Human Immunology. 2021;**82**(11):883-901. DOI: 10.1016/j.humimm.2021.07.009

[9] Morbe UM, Jorgensen PB, Fenton TM, et al. Human gut-associated lymphoid tissues (GALT); diversity, structure, and function. Mucosal Immunology. 2021;**14**(4):793-802. DOI: 10.1038/s41385-021-00389-4

[10] Stagg AJ. Intestinal dendritic cells in health and gut inflammation. Frontiers in Immunology. 2018;**9**:2883. DOI: 10.3389/fimmu.2018.02883

[11] Sun T, Nguyen A, Gommerman JL. Dendritic cell subsets in intestinal immunity and inflammation. Journal of Immunology. 2020;**204**(5):1075-1083. DOI: 10.4049/jimmunol.1900710

[12] Cheroutre H, Lambolez F, Mucida D. The light and dark sides of intestinal intraepithelial lymphocytes. Nature Reviews. Immunology. 2011;**11**(7):445-456. DOI: 10.1038/nri3007

[13] Han J, Liu N, Jin W, et al. TGF-beta controls development of TCRgammadelta(+)CD8alphaalpha(+) intestinal intraepithelial lymphocytes. Cell Discovery. 2023;**9**(1):52. DOI: 10.1038/s41421-023-00542-2

[14] Shi N, Li N, Duan X, et al. Interaction between the gut microbiome and mucosal immune system. Military Medical Research. 2017;**4**:14. DOI: 10.1186/s40779-017-0122-9

[15] Gunther C, Neumann H, Neurath MF, et al. Apoptosis, necrosis and necroptosis: Cell death regulation in the intestinal epithelium. Gut. 2013;**62**(7):1062-1071. DOI: 10.1136/gutjnl-2011-301364

[16] Brandtzaeg P, Pabst R. Let's go mucosal: Communication on slippery ground. Trends in Immunology. 2004;**25**(11):570-577. DOI: 10.1016/j.it.2004.09.005

[17] Olivares-Villagomez D, Van Kaer L. Intestinal intraepithelial lymphocytes: Sentinels of the mucosal barrier. Trends in Immunology. 2018;**39**(4):264-275. DOI: 10.1016/j.it.2017.11.003

[18] Ma H, Qiu Y, Yang H. Intestinal intraepithelial lymphocytes: Maintainers of intestinal immune tolerance and regulators of intestinal immunity. Journal of Leukocyte Biology. 2021;**109**(2):339-347. DOI: 10.1002/JLB.3RU0220-111

[19] Kc D, Sumner R, Lippmann S. Gut microbiota and health. Postgraduate Medicine. 2020;**132**(3):274. DOI: 10.1080/00325481.2019.1662711

[20] Bandeira A, Mota-Santos T, Itohara S, et al. Localization of gamma/delta T cells to the intestinal epithelium is independent of normal microbial colonization. The Journal of Experimental Medicine. 1990;**172**(1):239-244. DOI: 10.1084/jem.172.1.239

[21] Ostman S, Rask C, Wold AE, et al. Impaired regulatory T cell function in germ-free mice. European Journal of Immunology. 2006;**36**(9):2336-2346. DOI: 10.1002/eji.200535244

[22] Smith K, McCoy KD, Macpherson AJ. Use of axenic animals in studying the adaptation of mammals to their commensal intestinal microbiota. Seminars in Immunology. 2007;**19**(2):59-69. DOI: 10.1016/j.smim.2006.10.002

[23] Pickard JM, Zeng MY, Caruso R, et al. Gut microbiota: Role in pathogen colonization, immune responses, and inflammatory disease. Immunological Reviews. 2017;**279**(1):70-89. DOI: 10.1111/imr.12567

[24] Hapfelmeier S, Lawson MA, Slack E, et al. Reversible microbial colonization of germ-free mice reveals the dynamics of IgA immune responses. Science. 2010;**328**(5986):1705-1709. DOI: 10.1126/science.1188454

[25] Chung H, Pamp SJ, Hill JA, et al. Gut immune maturation depends on colonization with a host-specific microbiota. Cell. 2012;**149**(7):1578-1593. DOI: 10.1016/j.cell.2012.04.037

[26] Finnie IA, Dwarakanath AD, Taylor BA, et al. Colonic mucin synthesis is increased by sodium butyrate. Gut. 1995;**36**(1):93-99. DOI: 10.1136/gut.36.1.93

[27] Burger-van PN, Vincent A, Puiman PJ, et al. The regulation of intestinal mucin MUC2 expression by short-chain fatty acids: Implications for epithelial protection. The Biochemical Journal. 2009;**420**(2):211-219. DOI: 10.1042/BJ20082222

[28] Kayama H, Okumura R, Takeda K. Interaction between the microbiota, epithelia, and immune cells in the intestine. Annual Review of Immunology. 2020;**38**:23-48. DOI: 10.1146/annurev-immunol-070119-115104

[29] Chiu CY, Chan YL, Tsai MH, et al. Gut microbial dysbiosis is associated with allergen-specific IgE responses in young children with airway allergies. World Allergy Organization Journal. 2019;**12**(3):100021. DOI: 10.1016/j.waojou.2019.100021

[30] Meisel M, Mayassi T, Fehlner-Peach H, et al. Interleukin-15 promotes

intestinal dysbiosis with butyrate deficiency associated with increased susceptibility to colitis. The ISME Journal. 2017;**11**(1):15-30. DOI: 10.1038/ismej.2016.114

[31] Wang L, Zhu L, Qin S. Gut microbiota modulation on intestinal mucosal adaptive immunity. Journal of Immunology Research. 2019;**2019**:4735040. DOI: 10.1155/2019/4735040

[32] Weaver CT, Elson CO, Fouser LA, et al. The Th17 pathway and inflammatory diseases of the intestines, lungs, and skin. Annual Review of Pathology. 2013;**8**:477-512. DOI: 10.1146/annurev-pathol-011110-130318

[33] Cho H, Jaime H, de Oliveira RP, et al. Defective IgA response to atypical intestinal commensals in IL-21 receptor deficiency reshapes immune cell homeostasis and mucosal immunity. Mucosal Immunology. 2019;**12**(1):85-96. DOI: 10.1038/s41385-018-0056-x

[34] Moon C, Baldridge MT, Wallace MA, et al. Vertically transmitted faecal IgA levels determine extra-chromosomal phenotypic variation. Nature. 2015;**521**(7550):90-93. DOI: 10.1038/nature14139

[35] Brown EM, Kenny DJ, Xavier RJ. Gut microbiota regulation of T cells during inflammation and autoimmunity. Annual Review of Immunology. 2019;**37**:599-624. DOI: 10.1146/annurev-immunol-042718-041841

[36] Ma L, Morel L. Loss of gut barrier integrity In lupus. Frontiers in Immunology. 2022;**13**:919792. DOI: 10.3389/fimmu.2022.919792

[37] Barbhaiya M, Costenbader KH. Environmental exposures and the development of systemic lupus erythematosus. Current Opinion in Rheumatology. 2016;**28**(5):497-505. DOI: 10.1097/BOR.0000000000000318

[38] Wu Y, Wang CZ, Wan JY, et al. Dissecting the interplay mechanism between epigenetics and gut microbiota: Health maintenance and disease prevention. International Journal of Molecular Sciences. 2021;**22**(13):6933. DOI: 10.3390/ijms22136933

[39] Peng L, Li ZR, Green RS, et al. Butyrate enhances the intestinal barrier by facilitating tight junction assembly via activation of AMP-activated protein kinase in Caco-2 cell monolayers. The Journal of Nutrition. 2009;**139**(9):1619-1625. DOI: 10.3945/jn.109.104638

[40] Hsieh CY, Osaka T, Moriyama E, et al. Strengthening of the intestinal epithelial tight junction by Bifidobacterium bifidum. Physiological Reports. 2015;**3**(3):e12327. DOI: 10.14814/phy2.12327

[41] Mohd R, Chin S-F, Shaharir SS, et al. Involvement of gut microbiota in SLE and lupus nephritis. Biomedicine. 2023;**11**(3):653. DOI: 10.3390/biomedicines11030653

[42] Yaigoub H, Fath N, Tirichen H, et al. Bidirectional crosstalk between dysbiotic gut microbiota and systemic lupus erythematosus: What is new in therapeutic approaches? Clinical Immunology. 2022;**244**:109109. DOI: 10.1016/j.clim.2022.109109

[43] Mu Q, Kirby J, Reilly CM, et al. Leaky gut As a danger signal for autoimmune diseases. Frontiers in Immunology. 2017;**8**:598. DOI: 10.3389/fimmu.2017.00598

[44] Kyttaris VC, Juang YT, Tsokos GC. Immune cells and cytokines in systemic lupus erythematosus: An update.

Current Opinion in Rheumatology. 2005;**17**(5):518-522. DOI: 10.1097/01.bor.0000170479.01451.ab

[45] Zhou Z, Ding M, Huang L, et al. Toll-like receptor-mediated immune responses in intestinal macrophages; implications for mucosal immunity and autoimmune diseases. Clinical Immunology. 2016;**173**:81-86. DOI: 10.1016/j.clim.2016.09.005

[46] Kumar V. Corrigendum to 'Toll-like receptors in immunity and inflammatory diseases: Past, present, and future' [international Immunopharmacology 59 (2018) 391-412]. International Immunopharmacology. 2018;**62**:338. DOI: 10.1016/j.intimp.2018.06.044

[47] Mu Q, Zhang H, Luo XM. SLE: Another autoimmune disorder influenced by microbes and diet? Frontiers in Immunology. 2015;**6**:608. DOI: 10.3389/fimmu.2015.00608

[48] An J, Liu Y, Wang Y, et al. The role of intestinal mucosal barrier in autoimmune disease: A potential target. Frontiers in Immunology. 2022;**13**:871713. DOI: 10.3389/fimmu.2022.871713

[49] Pan F, Tang W, Zhou Z, et al. Intestinal macrophages in mucosal immunity and their role in systemic lupus erythematosus disease. Lupus. 2018;**27**(12):1898-1902. DOI: 10.1177/0961203318797417

[50] Crow MK. Pathogenesis of systemic lupus erythematosus: Risks, mechanisms and therapeutic targets. Annals of the Rheumatic Diseases. 2023;**82**(8):999-1014. DOI: 10.1136/ard-2022-223741

[51] Kim JW, Kwok SK, Choe JY, et al. Recent advances in our understanding of the link between the intestinal microbiota and systemic lupus erythematosus. International Journal of Molecular Sciences. 2019;**20**(19):4871. DOI: 10.3390/ijms20194871

[52] Roda G, Chien NS, Kotze PG, et al. Crohn's disease. Nature Reviews Disease Primers. 2020;**6**(1):22. DOI: 10.1038/s41572-020-0156-2

[53] Shouval DS, Rufo PA. The role of environmental factors in the pathogenesis of inflammatory bowel diseases: A review. JAMA Pediatrics. 2017;**171**(10):999-1005. DOI: 10.1001/jamapediatrics.2017.2571

[54] Ng SC, Shi HY, Hamidi N, et al. Worldwide incidence and prevalence of inflammatory bowel disease in the 21st century: A systematic review of population-based studies. Lancet. 2017;**390**(10114):2769-2778. DOI: 10.1016/S0140-6736(17)32448-0

[55] Ramos GP, Papadakis KA. Mechanisms of disease: Inflammatory bowel diseases. Mayo Clinic Proceedings. 2019;**94**(1):155-165. DOI: 10.1016/j.mayocp.2018.09.013

[56] Sanders ME, Merenstein DJ, Reid G, et al. Probiotics and prebiotics in intestinal health and disease: From biology to the clinic. Nature Reviews. Gastroenterology & Hepatology. 2019;**16**(10):605-616. DOI: 10.1038/s41575-019-0173-3

[57] Imhann F, Vich VA, Bonder MJ, et al. Interplay of host genetics and gut microbiota underlying the onset and clinical presentation of inflammatory bowel disease. Gut. 2018;**67**(1):108-119. DOI: 10.1136/gutjnl-2016-312135

[58] Morgan XC, Tickle TL, Sokol H, et al. Dysfunction of the intestinal microbiome in inflammatory bowel disease and treatment. Genome Biology. 2012;**13**(9):R79. DOI: 10.1186/gb-2012-13-9-r79

[59] Zhou L, Zhang M, Wang Y, et al. Faecalibacterium prausnitzii produces butyrate to maintain Th17/Treg balance and to ameliorate colorectal colitis by inhibiting histone deacetylase 1. Inflammatory Bowel Diseases. 2018;**24**(9):1926-1940. DOI: 10.1093/ibd/izy182

[60] Takeshita K, Mizuno S, Mikami Y, et al. A single species of clostridium subcluster XIVa decreased in ulcerative colitis patients. Inflammatory Bowel Diseases. 2016;**22**(12):2802-2810. DOI: 10.1097/MIB.0000000000000972

[61] Birrenbach T, Bocker U. Inflammatory bowel disease and smoking: A review of epidemiology, pathophysiology, and therapeutic implications. Inflammatory Bowel Diseases. 2004;**10**(6):848-859. DOI: 10.1097/00054725-200411000-00019

[62] Odenwald MA, Turner JR. The intestinal epithelial barrier: A therapeutic target? Nature Reviews. Gastroenterology & Hepatology. 2017;**14**(1):9-21. DOI: 10.1038/nrgastro.2016.169

[63] Kudelka MR, Stowell SR, Cummings RD, et al. Intestinal epithelial glycosylation in homeostasis and gut microbiota interactions in IBD. Nature Reviews. Gastroenterology & Hepatology. 2020;**17**(10):597-617. DOI: 10.1038/s41575-020-0331-7

[64] Gogokhia L, Buhrke K, Bell R, et al. Expansion of bacteriophages is linked to aggravated intestinal inflammation and colitis. Cell Host & Microbe. 2019;**25**(2):285-299. DOI: 10.1016/j.chom.2019.01.008

[65] Van der Sluis M, De Koning BA, De Bruijn AC, et al. Muc2-deficient mice spontaneously develop colitis, indicating that MUC2 is critical for colonic protection. Gastroenterology. 2006;**131**(1):117-129. DOI: 10.1053/j.gastro.2006.04.020

[66] Saez A, Gomez-Bris R, Herrero-Fernandez B, et al. Innate lymphoid cells in intestinal homeostasis and inflammatory bowel disease. International Journal of Molecular Sciences. 2021;**22**(14):7618. DOI: 10.3390/ijms22147618

[67] Mitsialis V, Wall S, Liu P, et al. Single-cell analyses of colon and Blood reveal distinct immune cell signatures of ulcerative colitis and Crohn's disease. Gastroenterology. 2020;**159**(2):591-608. DOI: 10.1053/j.gastro.2020.04.074

[68] Tindemans I, Joosse ME, Samsom JN. Dissecting the heterogeneity in T-cell mediated inflammation in IBD. Cell. 2020;**9**(1):110. DOI: 10.3390/cells9010110

[69] Rossen NG, Fuentes S, van der Spek MJ, et al. Findings from a randomized controlled trial of Fecal transplantation for patients with ulcerative colitis. Gastroenterology. 2015;**149**(1):110-118. DOI: 10.1053/j.gastro.2015.03.045

[70] Paramsothy S, Kamm MA, Kaakoush NO, et al. Multidonor intensive faecal microbiota transplantation for active ulcerative colitis: A randomised placebo-controlled trial. Lancet. 2017;**389**(10075):1218-1228. DOI: 10.1016/S0140-6736(17)30182-4

[71] Moayyedi P, Surette MG, Kim PT, et al. Fecal microbiota transplantation induces remission in patients with active ulcerative colitis in a randomized controlled trial. Gastroenterology. 2015;**149**(1):102-109. DOI: 10.1053/j.gastro.2015.04.001

[72] Vuyyuru SK, Kedia S, Kalaivani M, et al. Efficacy and safety of fecal transplantation versus targeted

therapies in ulcerative colitis: Network meta-analysis. Future Microbiology. 2021;**16**:1215-1227. DOI: 10.2217/fmb-2020-0242

[73] Narula N, Kassam Z, Yuan Y, et al. Systematic review and meta-analysis: Fecal microbiota transplantation for treatment of active ulcerative colitis. Inflammatory Bowel Diseases. 2017;**23**(10):1702-1709. DOI: 10.1097/MIB.0000000000001228

[74] Cheng F, Huang Z, Wei W, et al. Fecal microbiota transplantation for Crohn's disease: A systematic review and meta-analysis. Techniques in Coloproctology. 2021;**25**(5):495-504. DOI: 10.1007/s10151-020-02395-3

[75] Mayfield J. Diagnosis and classification of diabetes mellitus: New criteria. American Family Physician. 1998;**58**(6):1355-1362 1369-1370

[76] Han H, Li Y, Fang J, et al. Gut microbiota and type 1 diabetes. International Journal of Molecular Sciences. 2018;**19**(4):995. DOI: 10.3390/ijms19040995

[77] Zheng P, Li Z, Zhou Z. Gut microbiome in type 1 diabetes: A comprehensive review. Diabetes/Metabolism Research and Reviews. 2018;**34**(7):e3043. DOI: 10.1002/dmrr.3043

[78] Stojanovic I, Saksida T, Miljkovic D, et al. Modulation of intestinal ILC3 for the treatment of type 1 diabetes. Frontiers in Immunology. 2021;**12**:653560. DOI: 10.3389/fimmu.2021.653560

[79] Gulden E, Chao C, Tai N, et al. TRIF deficiency protects non-obese diabetic mice from type 1 diabetes by modulating the gut microbiota and dendritic cells. Journal of Autoimmunity. 2018;**93**:57-65. DOI: 10.1016/j.jaut.2018.06.003

[80] Niinisto S, Takkinen HM, Erlund I, et al. Fatty acid status in infancy is associated with the risk of type 1 diabetes-associated autoimmunity. Diabetologia. 2017;**60**(7):1223-1233. DOI: 10.1007/s00125-017-4280-9

[81] Tai N, Peng J, Liu F, et al. Microbial antigen mimics activate diabetogenic CD8 T cells in NOD mice. The Journal of Experimental Medicine. 2016;**213**(10):2129-2146. DOI: 10.1084/jem.20160526

[82] Burrows MP, Volchkov P, Kobayashi KS, et al. Microbiota regulates type 1 diabetes through toll-like receptors. Proceedings of the National Academy of Sciences of the United States of America. 2015;**112**(32):9973-9977. DOI: 10.1073/pnas.1508740112

[83] LeBlanc JG, Chain F, Martin R, et al. Beneficial effects on host energy metabolism of short-chain fatty acids and vitamins produced by commensal and probiotic bacteria. Microbial Cell Factories. 2017;**16**(1):79. DOI: 10.1186/s12934-017-0691-z

[84] Honda K, Littman DR. The microbiota in adaptive immune homeostasis and disease. Nature. 2016;**535**(7610):75-84. DOI: 10.1038/nature18848

[85] Ivanov II, Atarashi K, Manel N, et al. Induction of intestinal Th17 cells by segmented filamentous bacteria. Cell. 2009;**139**(3):485-498. DOI: 10.1016/j.cell.2009.09.033

[86] Gazali AM, Schroderus AM, Nanto-Salonen K, et al. Mucosal-associated invariant T cell alterations during the development of human type 1 diabetes. Diabetologia. 2020;**63**(11):2396-2409. DOI: 10.1007/s00125-020-05257-7

[87] Wong EB, Ndung'U T, Kasprowicz VO. The role of mucosal-associated invariant

T cells in infectious diseases. Immunology. 2017;**150**(1):45-54. DOI: 110.1111/imm.12673

[88] Dudakov JA, Hanash AM, van den Brink MR. Interleukin-22: Immunobiology and pathology. Annual Review of Immunology. 2015;**33**:747-785. DOI: 10.1146/annurev-immunol-032414-112123

[89] Rutz S, Wang X, Ouyang W. The IL-20 subfamily of cytokines--from host defence to tissue homeostasis. Nature Reviews. Immunology. 2014;**14**(12):783-795. DOI: 10.1038/nri3766

[90] Maxwell JR, Zhang Y, Brown WA, et al. Differential roles for Interleukin-23 and Interleukin-17 in intestinal Immunoregulation. Immunity. 2015;**43**(4):739-750. DOI: 10.1016/j.immuni.2015.08.019

[91] Lee JS, Tato CM, Joyce-Shaikh B, et al. Interleukin-23-independent IL-17 production regulates intestinal epithelial permeability. Immunity. 2015;**43**(4):727-738. DOI: 10.1016/j.immuni.2015.09.003

[92] Liang B, Wu C, Wang C, et al. New insights into bacterial mechanisms and potential intestinal epithelial cell therapeutic targets of inflammatory bowel disease. Frontiers in Microbiology. 2022;**13**:1065608. DOI: 10.3389/fmicb.2022.1065608

[93] Otte ML, Lama TR, Papapanagiotou J, et al. Mucosal healing and inflammatory bowel disease: Therapeutic implications and new targets. World Journal of Gastroenterology. 2023;**29**(7):1157-1172. DOI: 10.3748/wjg.v29.i7.1157

[94] Mougiakakos D, Kronke G, Volkl S, et al. CD19-targeted CAR T cells in refractory systemic lupus erythematosus. The New England Journal of Medicine. 2021;**385**(6):567-569. DOI: 10.1056/NEJMc2107725

[95] Xiao L, Van'T LB, van de Worp W, et al. Early-life nutritional factors and mucosal immunity in the development of autoimmune diabetes. Frontiers in Immunology. 2017;**8**:1219. DOI: 10.3389/fimmu.2017.01219

Chapter 3

Perspective Chapter: Specific Predictors of the Autoimmune Reactions Formation in Case of Immunocompetent Organs Damage in Patients with Myasthenia Gravis and Hepatosplenomegaly

Elena Klimova, Larisa Drozdova, Olena Lavinska, Sergey Sushkov and Valery Boyko

Abstract

The urgency of the problem is determined by the increasing prevalence and rapid progression of autoimmune diseases and autoimmune components in various nosologies. The aim is to study individual trigger factors, predictors of development, and the condition severity markers to substantiate complex treatment, including surgical tactics and the therapeutic target choice, in case of the immunocompetent organs (thymus and spleen) damage. In patients with myasthenia gravis the trigger markers were identified: the presence of herpes viruses persistence and mycoplasma; the relationship of certain human leucocyte antigen (HLA) molecules; high content of cytotoxic damage-associated molecular patterns (DAMPs); decreased expression of CD8+ T lymphocytes and co-stimulatory molecules CD3+CD4+CD28+. Some patients with myasthenia gravis had antibodies to α1 and α7 subunits nicotinic acetylcholine receptors (nAChR), etc. Patients with hepatosplenomegaly depending on the trigger factors (hepatitis HBV/HBC, herpes viruses (CMV/EBV)) and genetic predictors (hereditary enzymopathy) had specific markers, such as activation or inhibition of barrier function, reactive oxygen species (ROS) production, an increase in the concentration of cytokines, changes in the clusters of differentiation expression and specific autoantibodies. Thus, the creation of supplemented diagnostic protocols with additional markers for patients with various autoimmune reactions will make it possible to substantiate personalized immunocorrection.

Keywords: myasthenia gravis, hepatosplenomegaly, immunometabolic markers, autoantibodies, DAMPs, neutrophils phagocytic activity, surface receptors, cytokines

1. Introduction

There is an increase in autoimmune diseases and autoimmune component formation in the pathogenesis of many nosologies. The causes of autoimmune diseases are not completely clear. Many autoimmune diseases are multifactorial and with their progression, various organs can be involved in the pathological process [1].

The implementation of immune markers into clinical practice is limited due to insufficient information of the mechanisms that lead to changes in the metabolism of immune cells under the trigger factors.

Central and peripheral mechanisms of self-tolerance loss, genomic and epigenomic predictors associated with the autoimmune pathology (mutations of the autoimmune regulator (AIRE); HLA polymorphism; impaired editing of immunoglobulin genes; changes in the receptors structure and epigenomic marks formation of certain genes, etc.) are studied [2].

Some nosologies may have organ-nonspecific and organ-specific manifestations of reactions. If autoimmune disorders develop in the immune organs, then diseases are severe and often accompanied by life-threatening symptoms and a high risk of mortality. Such pathologies include generalized myasthenia gravis and hepatosplenomegaly, which are characterized by autoimmune damage of the immune organs: thymus and spleen, resulting in structural and functional disorders of these organs, in the form of hyperplasia or neoplasia. In autoimmune disorders of the thymus and spleen, it is relevant to investigate the features mechanisms formation of autoimmune reactions in patients with autoimmune myasthenia gravis and hepatosplenomegaly of various origins. It is necessary to search for additional pathogenetic links in order to develop approaches for diagnosing the mechanisms of formation and treatment of autoimmune reactions of various geneses [3].

Trigger factors for the occurrence of myasthenia gravis and hepatosplenomegaly can often be infectious factors, various specificities of autoantibodies, or stress factors that provoke the cells activation of the immune-neuroendocrine complex (e.g., with glandular syndrome). The most important predictor of the development of autoimmune diseases is a genetic predisposition. The relationship between the presence of certain HLA diplotypes and haplotypes is known; polymorphism of candidate genes that determine hereditary enzymopathy and high genome mutability; an increase in the frequency of chromosomal aberrations with certain clinical phenotypes of autoimmune diseases. Also, the formation of myasthenia gravis can occur as a result of epigenomic changes—hypermethylation of individual genes, which affects the synthesis of mRNA (inhibits or activates) responsible for the neurotransmitters production that affects the potential of the end plate. Myasthenia gravis is a disease with a progenitor course, characterized by progressive muscle weakness, ptosis, shortness of breath, and often the development of a myasthenic crisis with a fatal outcome [3, 4].

Hepatosplenomegaly accompanies different severe pathology, such as cirrhosis and hepatitis; and hereditary diseases such as Gaucher's syndrome, Pompe's syndrome, cystic fibrosis (associated with recurrent infectious and inflammatory processes), and other orphan diseases manifested by impaired hematopoiesis and osteogenesis. The progression of hepatosplenomegaly manifests itself in the form of portal hypertension and recurrent gastrointestinal bleeding, which is a risk factor for mortality. Recurrent bleeding in hepatosplenomegaly can be against the background of impaired blood flow in this area, and hypertension of the portal vein against the background of hypersplenism, as a result of hereditary pathology, in particular, lysosomal enzymopathy [1, 5]. It is also important to take into account violations of proliferation and differentiation of immunocompetent cells, due to changes in intercellular interaction and various humoral factors.

It is relevant to study the markers of the autoimmune pathologies development in order to determine specific therapeutic targets. The treatment of different autoimmune diseases is to relieve symptoms by suppressing the immune system. For this, hormone therapy, monoclonal antibodies, and plasmapheresis are used. But the treatment of these pathologies is not always effective. The treatment of myasthenia gravis and hepatosplenomegaly should take into account the multifactorial nature of nosologies with an autoimmune component. To achieve better results of complex treatment, it is necessary to study individual trigger factors, development predictors, and markers of the condition severity to assess the risk of mortality and disease progression. An effective method of providing urgent care for patients with myasthenia gravis and hepatosplenomegaly is surgery (removal of the thymus and spleen).

The aim is to study individual trigger factors, predictors of development, and the condition severity markers to substantiate complex treatment, including surgical tactics and the therapeutic target choice, in the case of the immunocompetent organs (thymus and spleen) damage.

2. Markers of self-tolerance loss in patients with various clinical forms of generalized myasthenia gravis

Myasthenia gravis is a multifactorial autoimmune disease characterized by pathological progressive muscle weakness. The violation of neuromuscular synaptic transmission is a basis of pathogenesis [6, 7]. The heterogeneity of the clinical forms of myasthenia gravis depends on a variety of pathogenetic mechanisms that are formed at various levels of the body's organization. Structural and functional disorders of the thymus are often manifested in autoimmune myasthenia gravis (in the form of hyperplasia or malignant thymoma) [8]. The pathogenetic development of myasthenia gravis is associated with the production of antibodies to the neuromuscular junction targets, to the structures of nicotinic acetylcholine receptors (nAChR), presynaptic ryanodine receptors (RyR), postsynaptic antigens – LRP4 (low-density lipoprotein receptor-related protein 4), agrin and tyrosine kinase receptors (MuSKR) [9–11]. Some authors have identified antibodies to extrasynaptic antigenic proteins—titin, actin, filamin, and actinin [12–14]. Depending on the presence of morphological and functional disorders of the thymus, myasthenia gravis is classified as thymus-independent or thymus-dependent (against the background of thymus hyperplasia or thymoma [15]. Neurotransmitter disorders in myasthenia gravis manifest themselves against the background of the self-tolerance loss to one's own tissues [16].

Myasthenia gravis is based on damaged mechanisms of immunological autotolerance. Normally, during the formation of central self-tolerance, a program for the development of lymphocytes is normally implemented, in which aggressive autoreactive clones are eliminated in the thymus. The AIRE complex is involved in the differentiation of thymocytes, migration and apoptosis within the thymus, alternative mRNA splicing, miRNA expression, transactivation of HLA expression, and is important for testing thymocyte autoreactivity [17]. Autoaggressive clones of T lymphocytes and B lymphocytes are formed in the central organs of the immune system in the central mechanisms of self-tolerance violation. Structural disorders in the thymus in myasthenia gravis may be the result of central self-tolerance loss due to impaired selection of autoreactive lymphocytes in the thymus. The mechanisms of peripheral self-tolerance loss may be formed due to a lack of AIRE gene expression in immunocompetent cells [18, 19]. The second way of self-tolerance formation is normally carried out in peripheral lymphoid organs and limits the activation of autoreactive lymphocytes with the help of T regulatory cells (Treg) that have not been eliminated by the mechanisms of central tolerance. These mechanisms ensure the peripheral tolerance formation [20].

Treatment of myasthenia gravis is determined by standard protocols and includes anticholinesterase drugs, corticosteroids, plasmapheresis, and surgical treatment—removal of the thymus. The whole complex of modern therapeutic approaches does not always achieve an acceptable effect [21, 22]. Removal of the thymus, the target of autoimmune aggression, does not always allow avoiding anticholinesterase drugs and sometimes leads to the development of myasthenic and cholinergic crises [23, 24]. A search is underway for new approaches in diagnostics for personalized treatment choice, taking into account immunocorrection.

2.1 Materials and methods in the study of immune reactions in myasthenia gravis

We examined 492 patients (18–78 years) with thymus-dependent and thymus-independent myasthenia gravis. The first group with thymus-independent myasthenia gravis included 241 patients aged 18–35 years (138 women and 103 men); the second group with thymus-dependent myasthenia gravis against the background of thymic hyperplasia consisted of 59 patients aged 36–72 years (44 women and 15 men), the third group with thymus-dependent myasthenia gravis and thymoma included 192 patients aged 35–78 years old (106 women and 86 men). The diagnosis was made on the basis of determining muscle weakness and pathological muscle fatigue, taking into account the temporal reversibility of clinical and electromyography changes. According to the indications, patients underwent thymectomy. Myasthenic crisis developed in 18% of patients with thymoma after surgery.

To assess the change in the spectrum of factors leading to impaired self-tolerance, a number of indicators characterizing genomic and epigenomic trigger factors that cause the development of myasthenia gravis were studied by the following methods:

- ELISA – the presence of viral persistence; concentration of total IgE; the cytokine profile IL-2, IL-4, IL-8, TNF-α; the presence of autoantibodies repertoire (the level of organ-specific antibodies, to cellular organelles (ANA), to α1 and α7 subunits of the nicotinic acetylcholine receptors (nAChR), and to the mitochondrial α7 subunit of neuronal nAChR in the thymus tissue).

- Light microscopy – leukocyte allele polymorphism class II antigens were assessed serologically using HLA phenotyping: DR1, DR2, DR3, DR5, DR7, DR52; the indicators of chemotaxis, adhesion and endocytosis of phagocytes in oxygen-independent phagocytosis.

- Fluorescence microscopy – the presence of autoantibodies ANA.

- Flow cytometry – the level of NK cells CD3-CD56+CD16+; B lymphocytes CD3-CD20+/CD45+, T helpers CD3+CD4+; cytotoxic T lymphocytes CD3+CD8+/CD45+; marker of early activation of the inflammatory process CD3+CD4+CD25+, regulatory T lymphocytes CD3+CD4+CD25+CD127-, costimulatory molecules CD3+CD4+CD28+, marker of late activation of lymphocytes (CD3+HLA-DR+).

The relative content of IgG class autoantibodies to 24 antigens of the main human organs and systems were studied in myasthenia gravis in blood serum samples: native DNA, Fc fragment of IgG (Fc), beta-2-glycoprotein I (β2), myocardial cell membrane antigens (CoM), myocardial β1-adrenergic receptors (βAR), platelet membrane antigens (TrM), vascular endothelial anionic proteins (ANCA), renal tissue cytoplasmic antigens (KiS), renal tissue membrane antigens (KiM), membrane lung tissue antigens (LuM), lung tissue cytoplasmic antigens (LuS), gastric mucosal cell membrane antigens (GaM), small intestine mucosal cell membrane antigens (ItM), liver tissue cytoplasmic antigens (HeS), liver cell mitochondrial antigens (HMMP), thyroglobulin (TG), thyroid stimulating hormone receptors (TSH-R), insulin (Ins), insulin receptors (Ins-R), adrenal cell membrane antigens (Adr), prostate and sperm cell membrane antigens (Spr), protein S100 (S100), astrocyte intermediate filament protein (GFAP), and myelin basic protein (MBP).

2.2 Trigger factors of autoimmune myasthenia gravis

Violation of molecular events that cause intercellular interactions during the development of an immune response to various infectious agents–PAMPs (pathogen-associated molecular patterns), endogenous and exogenous DAMPs (damage-associated molecular patterns), and food antigens can lead to a violation of the mechanisms of self-tolerance formation.

Long-term studies have shown that in patients with various clinical phenotypes of myasthenia gravis, immunoresistance disorders are interrelated with the accumulation of a combined antigenic load–a bacterial and viral infection (CMV, EBV, hepatitis virus HBV/HCV, herpes virus HSV-1, HSV-2, HHV-6, and mycoplasma).

Some food allergens and food-specific IgE and IgG4 also contribute to the increase in body allergic reactions and autoimmune component formation [25, 26].

2.2.1 Viral infection as a trigger factor for the development of myasthenia gravis

Trigger factors for dysfunction of the neuroendocrine-immune complex in myasthenia gravis can be exogenous stress factors, bacterial and viral infections in target organs, including the thymus, which change the activity of body cells and contribute to the development of long-term inflammation due to the presence of persister cells [27, 28].

A high titer of antibodies to CMV was revealed in myasthenia gravis and thymoma by 30 times and in the thymic hyperplasia by 23 times (**Figure 1A**).

The maximum incidence of CMV was in myasthenia gravis and thymoma–in 91.1% and 91.0%, respectively.

The titer of antibodies to EBV was significantly higher (by 10 times) than the reference values in all groups. The maximum concentration of antibodies to EBV was detected in thymic hyperplasia, and to CMV—in myasthenia gravis and thymoma (**Figure 1B**).

The highest incidence of antibodies to EBV was found in patients with thymic hyperplasia – in 100%. In myasthenia gravis and thymoma, the incidence of EBV was slightly lower and amounted to 89.0% and 87.4%, respectively.

Thus, the virus persistence can be considered as a trigger factor for this disease.

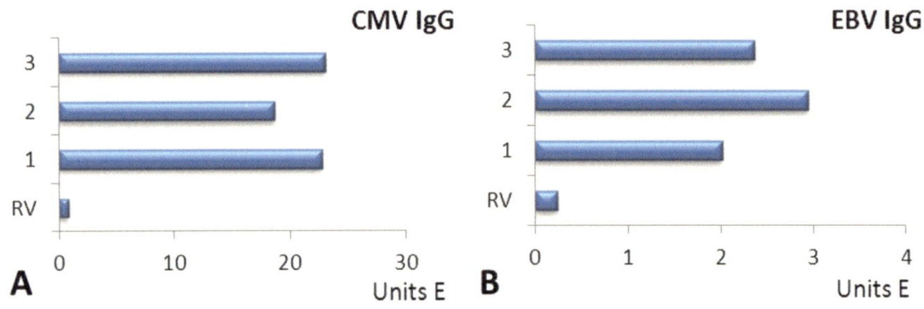

Figure 1.
The titer of IgG CMV (A) and IgG EBV (B) in patients with thymus-independent myasthenia gravis (1); thymus-dependent myasthenia gravis with thymic hyperplasia (2); thymus-dependent myasthenia gravis with thymoma (3); RV – Reference values.

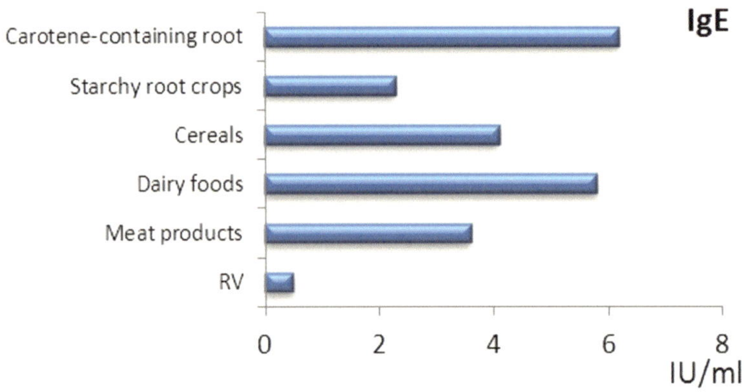

Figure 2.
The content of specific IgE antibodies to food allergens in patients with myasthenia gravis. RV – Reference values.

2.2.2 The content of total and allergen-specific IgE in patients with myasthenia gravis

In addition to infectious antigens, an exogenous trigger factor for the development of myasthenia gravis may be the presence of food allergens. We studied the concentration of total IgE in blood serum and allergen-specific IgE to food allergens in plasma. The panel of food allergens included antigens of animal proteins, cereals and flour, dairy products, mushrooms, nuts, carbohydrates, and drinks, in total 94 items.

In 72% of patients with generalized myasthenia gravis, congenital atopy was detected, as judged by an increased concentration of total IgE, which averaged 322.0 ± 34.0 IU/ml with a reference interval of 50–100 IU/ml.

In patients with myasthenia gravis, a high degree of polyclonal sensitization of allergen-specific IgE to foodstuffs in average 5.8 ± 0.6 IU/ml at reference values 0.30 ± 0.01 IU/ml of protein origin, cereals, and starch root crops containing carotenoids was revealed. Most often, sensitization to dairy products, to meat and cereals was detected in patients with myasthenia gravis (**Figure 2**).

In myasthenia gravis and thymoma, an increased content of specific IgE antibodies to dairy products (increase by 11 times), to meat products (increase by 7 times), to cereals (by 8 times), starch-containing root crops, to carotene-containing products relative to the reference values, with thymoma—to dairy and meat food allergens.

In some patients with polyclonal sensitization to food allergens, the concentration of total IgE did not exceed the reference values (from 70 to 130 IU/ml).

The absence of specific IgE in peripheral blood serum does not exclude the possibility of its participation in the pathogenesis of the IgE-dependent mechanism of allergic reactions, since its local synthesis or binding of synthesized IgE by tissues is possible, which can occur without changing the concentration of IgE in peripheral blood [29].

Thus, one of the possible epigenomic factors in the formation of autoimmune myasthenia gravis may be food allergy.

2.3 Dysregulation of immunoreactivity and changes in the cytokine profile in different clinical phenotypes of myasthenia gravis

The activation of numerous and specialized immune cell subpopulations are under the control of the cellular regulation and cytokine network. Secondary activation of the expression of mitochondrial and nuclear genes is carried out by PAMPs (pathogen-associated molecular patterns) and DAMPs (damage-associated molecular patterns), which contribute to the synthesis of cytokines, nucleotides, nucleosides, RNA, and heat shock molecules [30]. The identified infectious trigger factors leading to the formation of molecular compounds PAMPs also contribute to the formation of various classes of endogenous cytotoxic molecules DAMPs, related to immunogenic molecules that are formed as a result of the breakdown of necrotic and apoptotic cells, as well as cells undergoing autophagy.

We revealed an increase of the IFN-γ content in all groups. The maximum increase in the IFN-γ concentration was observed in thymic hyperplasia.

In thymic hyperplasia and thymoma IL-4 content exceeded the reference values. The maximum value of IL-4 was found in thymoma – 66.4 ± 4.5 pg./ml; in thymic hyperplasia, this cytokine was increased sevenfold to 49.2 ± 5.2 pg./ml (**Figure 3**).

Patients with thymoma had the maximum increase in IL-8. According to most authors, IL-8 manifests itself as a factor in enhancing tumor progression. This is explained by the action of IL-8 as an autocrine tumor growth factor and as a factor in enhancing angiogenesis by influencing the capillaries of metastases [22].

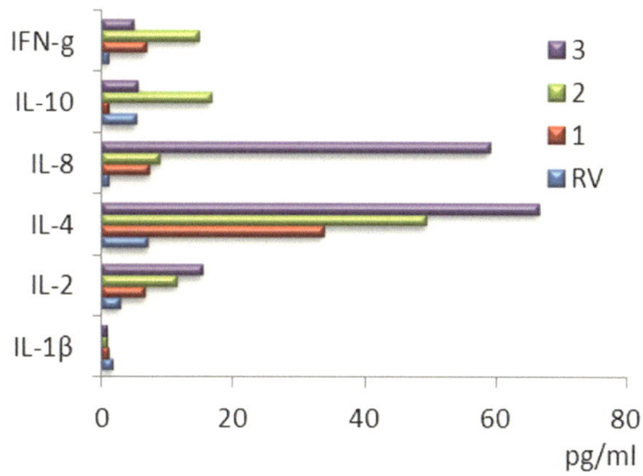

Figure 3.
The contents of cytokines in patients with thymus-independent myasthenia gravis (1); thymus-dependent myasthenia gravis with thymic hyperplasia (2); thymus-dependent myasthenia gravis with thymoma and (3); RV – Reference values.

Synthesis of IL-10 was inhibited in the myasthenia gravis and amounted to 1.0 ± 0.6 pg./ml and in the thymoma – 5.5 ± 0.9 pg./ml. In the thymic hyperplasia, IL-10 was maximally elevated and exceeded reference values by three times.

The maximum increase (up to 15.3 ± 0.4 pg./ml) in IL-2 was revealed in thymoma.

IL-2 is an inducer of all cytotoxic cells that takes part in the formation of the Th1 phenotype and increases the production of IFN-γ. The synthesis of IL-2 forms the affinity of the TCR and activates HLA molecules. An increase of IL-2 was observed in the thymic hyperplasia and thymoma.

Thus, the most significant changes were found in the content of IL-4, IL-8, and IL-2.

2.4 An additional target of autoimmunization is the presence of nAChR in thymus mitochondria in patients with thymoma

In the literature, changes in the thymus are practically not described, although there is a concept about the leading role of impaired central differentiation of T lymphocytes. Together with Professor Skok M.V. (Laboratory of Immunology cell receptors of the O.V. Palladin Institute of Biochemistry of the National Academy of Sciences of Ukraine) studies were carried out on the presence of α7 subunits of neuronal nicotinic acetylcholine receptors (nAChR) in mitochondria of thymus different layers obtained from patients with thymic hyperplasia and thymoma.

A significant difference was found in the content of α7 neuronal nAChR of thymus mitochondria in patients with thymic hyperplasia and thymoma (**Figure 4A**). The level of α7 neuronal nAChR mitochondria in the thymus in patients with thymic hyperplasia was 0.23 units E and in thymoma – 0.43 units E, which was 1.9 times higher than in thymus mitochondria not affected by the tumor process (**Figure 4A**).

The function of nAChRs in mitochondria is to control the formation of the mitochondrial transient conduction pore, which is the source of proapoptotic factors and reactive oxygen species (ROS) released in the cytosol (**Figure 4B**) [31, 32]. From this, it follows that the revealed difference between the mitochondria of patients with and without thymoma indicates that tumor transformation is accompanied by an increase in mitochondrial nAChRs, and this maintains the viability of tumor cells.

The presence of the α7 subunit nAChR in thymus mitochondria suggested that this structure can also serve as an additional target for inducing the formation of

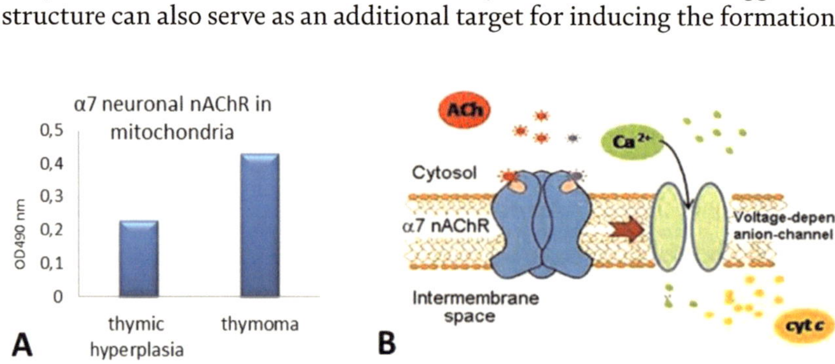

Figure 4.
Changes in α7 nAChR level mitochondria in patients with thymic hyperplasia and thymoma (A) and the scheme of α7 neuronal nAChR localization and functioning in the outer membrane of mitochondria (B); adapted from [31].

autoantibodies. Specific autoantibodies can bind to certain domains—subunits of nAChR and cause destruction of these receptors in the thymus.

2.5 Specific markers of self-tolerance loss in various clinical phenotypes of myasthenia gravis

The frequency of occurrence of autoantibodies to the α1 subunit of nicotinic acetylcholine receptors (nAChR) in all groups was 100% higher than the reference values.

Patients with thymic hyperplasia had the maximum increase (by 2.2 times) of antibodies to the α1 subunit nAChR.

The frequency of occurrence of antibodies to the α7 subunit nAChR was only in 20% of cases higher than in the control comparison group.

Patients with myasthenia gravis had the maximum increase (1.9 times) in antibodies to the α7 subunit nAChR.

2.5.1 The autoantibodies spectrum to various targets in various clinical phenotypes of myasthenia gravis

Patients with myasthenia gravis and thymoma had the widest range of autoantibodies (AABs)—12 and 11 specificities out of 24 studied, respectively.

Patients with thymic hyperplasia had 6 specificities out of 24 researched.

Four specificities of autoantibodies were detected with high frequency in all forms of myasthenia gravis: AABs to the TSH receptor (myasthenia gravis—with a frequency of 55.6%, thymic hyperplasia—66.7%, thymoma—70%), to thyroglobulin (myasthenia gravis—33.3%, thymic hyperplasia—66.7%, thymoma—40%), to β2-glycoprotein I (myasthenia gravis—33.3%, thymic hyperplasia—33.3%, thymoma—20%) and to hepatocyte mitochondria (myasthenia gravis—55.6%, thymic hyperplasia—33.3%, thymoma—10%). In all patients, organ-specific AABs at different levels were detected with different frequency (from 33 to 56%) (**Figure 5**).

Thus, in patients with myasthenia gravis and thymoma, the same additional targets for AABs were identified: membrane antigens of the mucous cells membrane of the stomach and small intestine, membrane and cytoplasmic antigens of the lung tissue, which may indicate possible identical mechanisms for the formation of myasthenia gravis these forms.

The progression of myasthenia gravis in ontogenesis may lead to the formation of myasthenia gravis on the background of thymoma in elderly patients. In myasthenia gravis with elevated concentrations of autoantibodies in the gastric mucosa (parietal cells), the presence of food allergy (high concentration of specific IgG4 and IgE) was revealed as a possible pathogenetic factor in the development of this disease.

Organ-specific antibodies in patients with thymic hyperplasia had other cellular targets and were represented by the following localization: AABs to insulin protein and astrocytes. In addition, in thymic hyperplasia, the concentration of AABs to the TSH receptor and thyroglobulin significantly exceeded the content of these antibodies in the myasthenia gravis and thymoma.

In patients with myasthenia gravis and thymoma, the concentration of autoantibodies to β2-glycoprotein I was significantly higher than in the patients with thymic hyperplasia.

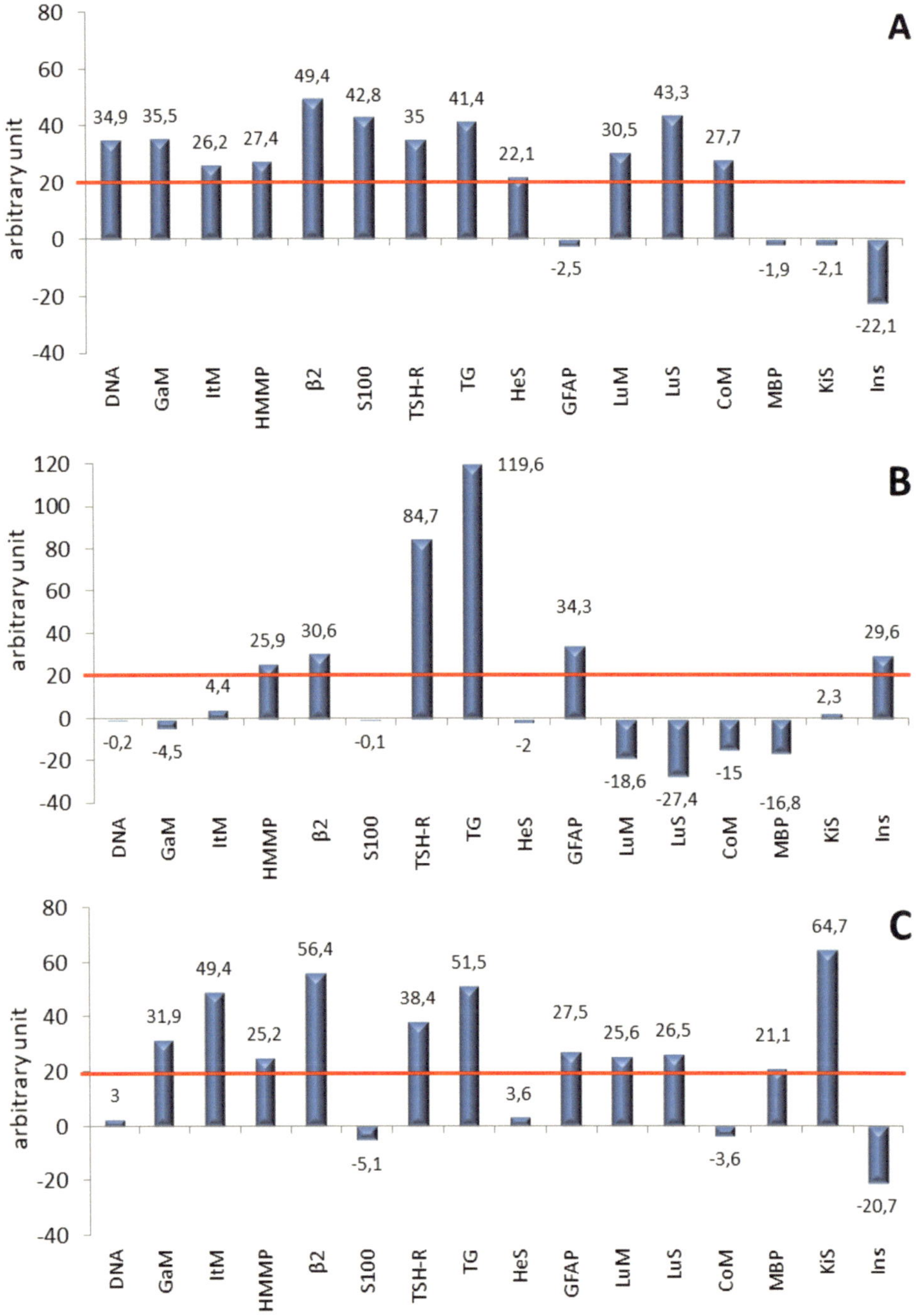

Figure 5.
Change in the relative autoantibodies content from the individual average level of immunoreactivity (red line) in patients with myasthenia gravis (A), thymic hyperplasia (B), and thymoma (C).

The selective rise in the level of relative immunoreactivity in reaction with the above antigens can be considered as a factor in existing or emerging disorders in the relevant organs and systems.

2.6 Relationship of class II HLA various alleles antigens with different clinical phenotypes of myasthenia gravis

In addition to trigger exogenous factors identified in the examined patients with myasthenia gravis, the assessment of leukocyte antigens of class II HLA (Human Leukocyte Antigens) revealed the relationship between certain HLA DR alleles. HLA molecules play a central role in the immune response, determining the severity and direction of the reactions to antigenic exposure by forming a macromolecular complex of recognized antigens (HLA and T-cell receptor TCR) [33]. Many mononucleotide differences in the HLA genes determine their polymorphic variants. Some alleles may be associated with the development of certain pathological conditions, such as endocrine, reproductive, thrombolytic, and cardiovascular. Expression of HLA molecules on the immune system cell surface is a complex dynamic process, on which their functional activity largely depends [34].

In patients with a genetic predisposition the pathological activation of the immune system is associated with the functioning of the HLA-antigen complex, and it leads to the autoimmune disease development [35]. HLA-B27 heavy chains can bind to innate immune receptors on natural killer NK cells [36, 37].

The polymorphism of the HLA genes determines the selection of T lymphocytes during maturation in the thymus. In the presence of certain alleles of the HLA system genes, the elimination of T lymphocytes, which carry receptors for certain autoantigens on their surface, is impaired, while in a healthy body such T lymphocytes are destroyed at the maturation [38]. The function of class II HLA receptors is to present antigen peptides from the extracellular space. Pathological activation of the immune system in patients with a genetic predisposition can lead to autoimmune processes and a severe course of other diseases and a negative prognosis.

We revealed the presence of various allelic phenotypes of HLA associated with various forms of myasthenia gravis. Among the entire cohort of patients, the HLA DR5 phenotype was the most common.

In patients with myasthenia gravis, the allele encountered with the maximum frequency revealed HLA DR5 and HLA DR2.

In patient with thymic hyperplasia the phenotypes HLA DR5 (in 70%) and HLA DR1 (in 60%) were detected with high frequency.

In patients with thymoma, the frequency of occurrence for the HLA DR7 allele was revealed. In locally advanced thymomas, HLA DR3 and HLA DR52 were also detected.

Thus, a high frequency of detection of the HLA DR5 allele, both in homozygous and heterozygous states, was shown in all patients.

Patients with thymoma had high frequency of HLA DR7. The presence of this allele can serve as a diagnostic and prognostic marker for the thymoma development in patients included in cohort with myasthenia gravis without thymoma and also have the HLA DR7 allele.

2.7 Expression of cell surface clusters differentiation on lymphocytes in myasthenia gravis

To assess the effectiveness of interaction between T cells and B cells during the immune response development to various thymus-dependent bacterial and viral antigens, the expression of different subpopulation of lymphocytes was determined.

In 45% of patients with various phenotypes of myasthenia gravis, a decrease in CD8+ expression was noted.

An increase in aggressive clones' natural killers CD3-CD56+CD16+ was revealed against the background of a decrease in cytotoxic CD8+. And it can lead to excessive cytotoxicity.

Patients with myasthenia gravis had the minimum level (38.4%) of CD4+CD28+ expression.

In patients with thymic hyperplasia, CD4+CD28+ expression was 1.2 times higher than in myasthenia gravis.

Patients with thymoma had the greatest increase (54.3%) in positive CD4+CD28+ cells.

In 18% of the patients, there was a decrease in the expression of CD8+ and CD4+CD28+.

Patients with myasthenia gravis and thymoma had a fourfold decrease in the expression of CD25+ on CD4+ T cells compared to the reference values (**Figure 6**).

Patients with thymic hyperplasia had the level of CD4+CD25+ cells on average 30% lower than reference values (**Figure 6**).

Probably, in thymoma, CD4+ T cells with a high expression of the CD25 molecule predominated, since it is these cells that have suppressor activity [39].

A significant increase in the lymphocytes late activation marker (CD3+HLA-DR+) was revealed in thymic hyperplasia (by 34%) and thymoma (by 87%) groups.

Violation of molecular processes that determine intercellular interactions during the development of an immune response to various infectious agents can lead to disruption of the mechanisms of self-tolerance formation [40].

2.8 The content of antinuclear autoantibodies (ANA) in patients with thymoma

It was revealed the presence of antinuclear autoantibodies (ANA, ELISA method) in patients with locally advanced thymoma (who developed myasthenic crisis in the postoperative period), the content of which was four times higher than the reference level and averaged 4.2 ± 0.2 units.

In myasthenia gravis and thymic hyperplasia ANA was not detected in the blood serum.

To visualize the specificity of ANA, immunofluorescent analysis was performed, which made it possible to identify targets for autoantibodies (AABs) in the form of various components of cell nuclei in patients with thymoma—ANA to histones,

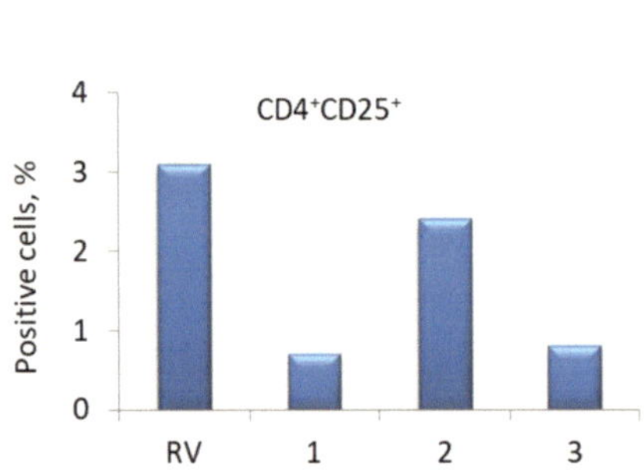

Figure 6.
Expression of CD4+CD25+ in patients with various types of self-tolerance loss: 1 – Myasthenia gravis; 2 – Thymic hyperplasia; and 3 – Thymoma; RV – Reference values.

double-stranded DNA, and other chromatin-associated antigens (**Figure 7A**). Since due to the action of various factors, reparative processes in DNA are disrupted, a lot of erroneous codes appear in the structure of the DNA helix, which upon the next reading triggers the disturbed mechanism of histone formation.

In patients with lymphoepithelial thymoma, ANA to chromosome centromeres was detected (**Figure 7B**). Centromeres play an important role in the regulation and functioning of the cell cycle. Ordered linkage and separation of centromeres is a prerequisite for the normal distribution of chromosomes in a mitotic cell. Violation of this due to the presence of antibodies leads to chromosomal instability and cancerous transformation.

Also, patients with thymoma had ANA to the centromeric protein F (CTNPF) (**Figure 7C**); to the protein involved in the formation of the mitotic spindle (NuMa), which is associated with the centrosome (**Figure 7D**); to the MSA-2 antigen of mitotic spindle fibers (**Figure 7E**), which is involved in the regulation of transcription during the G1/S transition of the mitotic cell cycle; to the cytoskeleton, represented by proteins cytokeratins and tropomyosin (**Figure 7F**).

It is known that cytokeratins are part of the intermediate filaments of the cell cytoskeleton, and tropomyosin is a fibrous protein that interacts with actin in muscle tissue and is involved in the process of muscle contraction.

2.9 Changes in immunoreactivity and structural organization of the thymus during the development of the immunopathological process with various types of self-tolerance loss in myasthenia gravis

There is a self-sustaining immune response to self-antigens in myasthenia gravis, which leads to cell damage. The study of the self-tolerance loss mechanisms in myasthenia gravis is of fundamental and practical importance; it can be used to predict the course of the disease and select treatment tactics.

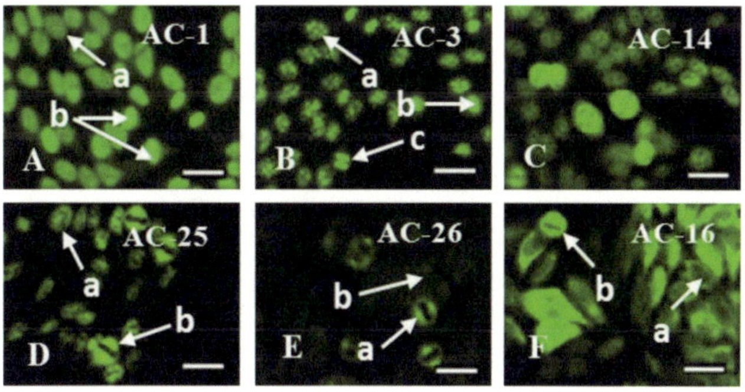

Figure 7.
Antinuclear autoantibodies (ANA) in myasthenia associated with thymoma: A – To histones and double-stranded DNA (a – Stained nucleoli, b – Mitotic cells); B – To the centromeres (a – Uniform distribution of granules in the nucleus, b – Metaphase stage, c – Anaphase stage); C – To centromeric protein F (CTNPF); D – To the achromatin spindle protein NuMa (a – no staining of the nucleoli, b - fluorescence of the achromatin spindle fibers); E – To the MSA-2 antigen of mitotic spindle fibers (a – Mitotic spindle fibers, b – Unstained nuclei of interphase cells); F – To cytoskeletal proteins (a – Microtubules and intermediate fibers, b – Cytoskeletal proteins in mitotic cells). Fluorescent microscopy. Scale bar 20 µm. Codes AC (AC – Anti-cell pattern) in accordance with the international consensus on ANA patterns (ICAP) are presented. FITC staining of HEp-2 standard antigenic substrates after interaction with serum antibodies; magnification ×1000.

A range of trigger factors for myasthenia gravis, thymic hyperplasia, and thymoma, such as persistence infection and IgG4 and IgE antibodies to food antigens was determined.

Various clinical types of myasthenia gravis have relationship with specific HLA alleles. Patients with myasthenia gravis had the highest frequency of occurrence of the HLA DR5 and HLA DR2 allele. In thymic hyperplasia, in addition to the HLA DR5 allele, the HLA DR1 allele was found with a high frequency. Patients with thymoma had a high frequency of HLA DR7 and HLA DR2 alleles.

In 50% of all patients, a decrease in the subpopulation of T killer cells CD8+ and an increase in NK cells CD3-CD56+CD16+ were observed.

Violation of dual recognition by changing the expression of CD4+CD28+ led to a violation of peripheral self-tolerance.

Patients with myasthenia gravis had the minimum level of CD4+CD28+ expression.

Patients with thymoma had the maximum increase in CD4+CD28+ cells.

In myasthenia gravis and thymoma was a fourfold decrease in the early marker of the inflammatory response CD4+CD25+.

In thymic hyperplasia and thymoma was a significant increase in the marker of lymphocytes late activation CD3+HLA-DR+.

Peripheral disorders of humoral self-tolerance in the form of an increase in the concentration of various autoantibodies were detected in most patients with myasthenia gravis, thymic hyperplasia, and thymoma. Autoantibodies react with cell surface molecules and have both blocking and stimulating effects (depending on the features of the target molecule and the signaling pathways associated with it).

An increase in the concentration of autoantibodies to the α1 subunit of nicotinic acetylcholine receptors (nAChRs) was shown in all patients.

The α7 subunit of neuronal nAChRs is an additional target for inducing the formation of autoantibodies mitochondrial structures. Mitochondria of thymocytes in patients with thymoma had the maximum level of α7 nAChR.

In addition to nAChR antibodies, a wide range of organ-specific antibodies were detected in all patients: out of 24 antigenic specificities of the panel, autoimmune antibodies were detected to 16. For all examined patients with myasthenia gravis (myasthenia gravis, thymic hyperplasia, and thymoma) is characterized by the presence of a high titer of autoantibodies to the TSH receptor and thyroglobulin, to hepatocyte mitochondria and β2-glycoprotein I.

Young patients with myasthenia gravis and elderly patients with thymoma had autoantibodies to the same targets (membrane antigens of mucous membrane cells stomach and small intestine, membrane and cytoplasmic antigens of lung tissue).

In addition to the main four antigenic targets characteristic of all group' patients with thymic hyperplasia also formed an organ-specific antibodies to other targets: the insulin protein and the protein of astrocyte intermediate filaments.

Only patients with thymoma had antinuclear antibodies (ANA): to histones and double-stranded DNA, to chromosomal centromere proteins, to centromeric protein F (CTNPF), to the achromatin spindles protein NuMa, to the mitotic spindle fiber antigen MSA-2, to cytoskeletal proteins.

Perhaps the reason for the diversity of antibodies is a violation of the negative selection of autoreactive T lymphocytes and the presentation of self-antigens. The detection of autoantibodies with different characteristics in the blood serum of patients with myasthenia gravis proves the immunological heterogeneity of this disease and the different mechanisms of self-tolerance loss.

The results of some regularity in the autoimmune pathology formation make it possible to determine additional targeted for their treatment. The prognosis of myasthenia gravis progression and remission development can be carried out using the identified markers of self-tolerance loss. Specialists of the Institute (State Institution "Zaycev V. T. Institute of General and Urgent Surgery of National Academy of Medical Sciences of Ukraine) carried out the complex treatment in patients with myasthenia gravis, thymic hyperplasia, and thymoma, perform thymectomy in patients with thymic hyperplasia and locally advanced thymoma. Treatment methods are used in various combinations and sequences in patients with thymoma (embolization of thymus vessels in order to reduce the tumor size; endovascular transcatheter sclerotherapy in patients with locally advanced thymoma in the superior vena cava syndrome with transvenous destruction of the thymus parenchyma as a preoperative preparation). Thymomectomy and thymectomy often lead to the development of postoperative complications in the form of myasthenic and cholinergic crises (**Figure 8**).

Indications for surgical treatment of thymoma are close to absolute, but as a rule, without taking into account the course nature and the disease severity.

In 12% young patients with progressive myasthenia gravis, surgical treatment is indicated.

Determination of immunological markers in myasthenia gravis made it possible to substantiate new approaches to treatment in young patients with myasthenia gravis.

In elderly patients with locally advanced thymoma, it is necessary to reduce the tumor volume *via* applying new X-ray endovascular interventions.

But, unfortunately, surgical treatment of patients with thymoma leads to satisfactory remission only in a third of patients, since it basically eliminates some of the disease symptoms.

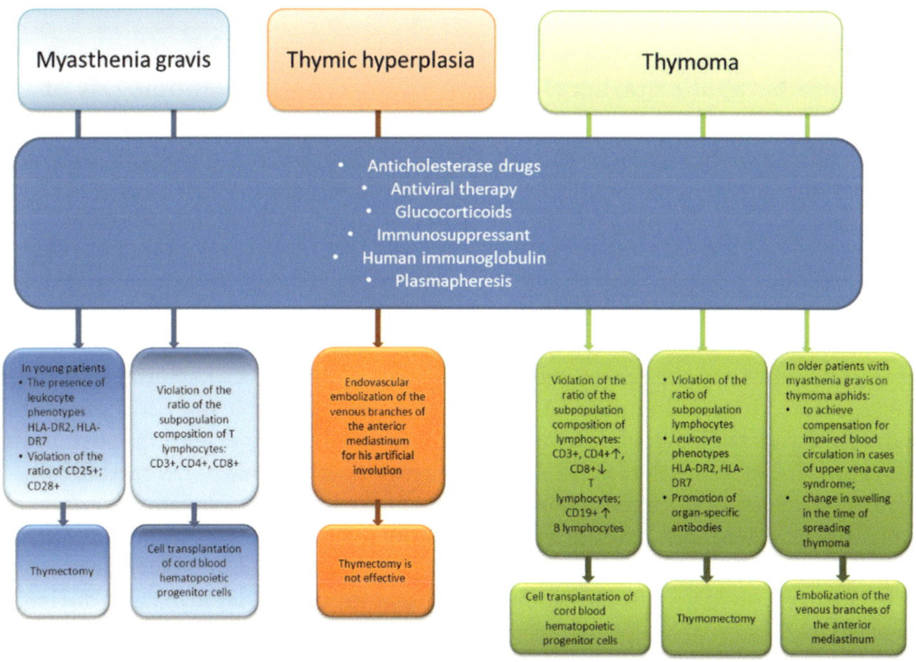

Figure 8.
The strategy of treatment for patients with myasthenia gravis.

The age-dependent development of the disease is not always taken into account for choosing treatment tactics. It has been shown that the disease onset in young patients with myasthenia gravis is often characterized by a low degree of severity.

The progression of myasthenia gravis in ontogenesis can lead to myasthenia gravis and thymic hyperplasia in elderly patients. In this case, surgical treatment is not effective and can lead to complications and death [41, 42].

If genetic predictors of HLA DR2, HLA DR7, and markers of central autotolerance loss are detected in young patients with myasthenia gravis, then it is advisable to recommend thymectomy in the early stages of the disease. This is necessary to avoid further thymus-dependent myasthenia gravis, in the form of locally advanced thymomas and postoperative complications during surgical intervention at a later stage of the disease—an attack of autoantibodies on other target organs, bleeding.

If markers of peripheral autotolerance loss are detected in patients with myasthenia gravis (possible thymus hyperplasia formation), then thymectomy is not advisable.

We also have a positive experience in the complete cure of generalized myasthenia gravis in non-operated patients after a long 35-day fast followed by stimulation of the phagocytic function of neutrophils (since their endoitosis, according to our data, was suppressed in all patients with myasthenia gravis [43]) using a composite preparation containing enzymes.

It is relevant to determine additional markers in patients with myasthenia gravis, thymic hyperplasia, and thymoma, leading to changes in the afferent and efferent links of immunity for complex treatment, including targeted immunocorrection.

Individual methods of correction for self-tolerance loss in myasthenia gravis should take into account the state of the immunity main organ and include the use of diet, immunosuppressants, specific neutralizing immunoglobulins, massive IgG therapy, and the use of anti-inflammatory recombinant interleukins.

3. Immunometabolic markers in patients with hepatosplenomegaly of various etiologies

An enlarged spleen is often combined with liver pathology. Both organs are involved in the pathological process, and hepatosplenomegaly (or hepatolienal syndrome) develops. Hepatosplenomegaly (HSM) accompanies a number of pathological conditions (hepatitis cirrhosis, parasitic lesions, storage diseases, malignant and benign tumors, acute and chronic diseases) and is often complicated by portal hypertension, recurrent bleeding from esophageal varices. Causes of enlargement of the spleen, indicating the presence of hepatolienal syndrome are bacterial infections, protozoal infections, helminthiases, immune thrombocytopenic purpura, splenogenic neutropenia, agranulocytosis, polyarthritis nodosa, portal hypertension, portal vein occlusion, Nimmann-Pick disease, Gaucher disease, Felty's syndrome, sarcaidosis, amyloidosis, hepatocerebral dystrophy, and mononucleosis [5]. Hepatosplenomegaly disrupts the main function of the spleen to eliminate defective senescent cells (that have changed their phenotype) and PAMPs (pathogen-associated molecular patterns) [44]. The liver mediates detoxification reactions at the molecular level, and during infection, pathological molecular processes occur with the formation of cytotoxic molecular patterns of cellular debris (DAMPs—damage-associated molecular patterns) [45, 46]. Thus, it is necessary for additional screening and differential diagnosis of hepatolienal syndrome.

3.1 Trigger factors in the development of hepatosplenomegaly

Hepatosplenomegaly trigger factors are infectious antigens in the form of PAMPs viral structures of microorganisms and protozoa [30, 47]. The study of the bacterial contamination degree and viral load in patients with HSM are contradictory. It is considered that viral hepatitis and alcohol are trigger factors for the development of a HSM complicated course. Alcohol and infectious antigens exacerbate the development of hepatomegaly [48, 49]. However, there is a pronounced clinical heterogeneity of etiological factors and features of reactions occurring in the liver and spleen under the influence of other triggers and predictors [50, 51]. In this work, the studies made it possible to identify trigger factors, as well as genetic predictors in the form of specific immunological and metabolic markers for HSM development.

3.2 Bacterial and viral persisters of hepatosplenomegaly

There is a long-term presence of infectious antigens in accordance with the hypothesis of hidden antigens, the presence of superantigens, molecular mimicry, antigen complementarity, and idiotype-antiidypic interactions [52]. Against the background of immunosuppression, viral and bacterial persistent cells can form, which generates irreversible inflammatory reactions. These contribute to the development of irreversible autoimmune pathologies, including in hepatosplenomegaly [53, 54]. In prolonged persistent infection, the spectrum of specific T lymphocytes and antibodies expands, and more and more new epitopes of the same protein or new proteins can be recognized [55]. And here there is a risk that some of the lymphocytes will be able to react with their own antigens, eventually leading to autoimmune disorders. This is especially true for persistent infections and the release of self-proteins, which leads to the development of an immune response against self-epitopes [52]. In the case of immunosuppression of innate and adaptive immunity due to the relationship of infection with immunocompetent cells, the existing basic postulates were expanded with additional markers. Today, the relationship of infectious agents with 30 autoimmune diseases has been established [56, 57].

3.3 Structural and functional features of the hepatobiliary system organs to trigger factors

During the immune reactions formation in response to various antigens in the spleen and liver, activation and redistribution of cellular elements occur, which affects their mass, size, and function. Morphological and functional changes in the spleen also depend on the migratory properties of immunocompetent cells in the spleen compartments. Infectious antigens change the profile of immune cells. The spleen accumulates activated macrophages expressing CD68 receptors; CD4 and CD8 T lymphocytes; CD20 B lymphocytes; CD57 NK cells, which should normally leave the spleen [58]. Immune cells change phenotype and move to the spleen in accordance with the stages of the immune response. The spleen, in addition to activating macrophages and differentiating lymphoid cells, takes part in the formation of antibodies, also destroys erythrocytes and platelets, synthesizes mediators that affect hematopoiesis in the bone marrow, and ensures the maturation of immunocompetent cells [59]. Hyperplasia of the spleen develops with an increase in the phagocytic function of the spleen against the background of autoimmune diseases. The spleen increases against the background of inflammation associated with a violation of the immune system.

The presence of an immune response directed against antigens or self-tissues may be a primary independent process in relation to tissue damage. Enlargement of the spleen can be the cause of hypersplenism, that is, sequestration and high destruction of blood cells of two or more cell lines by splenic macrophages. In hypersplenism, cytopenia is observed, and in the bone marrow— enhanced hematopoiesis [44].

The liver contains resident immunocompetent cells, hepatic stellate cells (Ito cells), and resident macrophages (Kupffer cells), which are actively involved in changing the functional state of hepatocytes [60, 61]. Ito cells can induce the development of liver fibrosis under the influence of exogenous factors [62]. Activated fibroblasts act as producers of excess collagen. Fat-storing Ito cells transform into myoblasts and synthesize extracellular collagen. In response to damage by antigens, Kupffer cells produce pro-inflammatory cytokines, which are an additional factor in apoptosis and autophagy of hepatocytes against the background of a large amount of reactive oxygen species (ROS) production. It is the cytokine-producing Kupffer cells that are the activators of this negative process [63, 64].

3.4 Materials and methods in the study of immunological reactions in hepatosplenomegaly

We examined 148 patients with hepatosplenomegaly (HSM), age 22–71 years. Patients, depending on the severity, underwent sclerotherapy of esophageal varices; embolization of the splenic and left gastric arteries, and other methods of surgical treatment. Depending on the etiological factors, all patients with HSM were divided into three groups.

The first group (I) included 74 patients with cirrhosis of the liver against the background of the hepatitis virus, of which 60 people (34 men and 26 women) aged 22 to 71 years with cirrhosis of the liver against the background of the hepatitis C virus (HCV), 6 men aged 49 to 68 years with cirrhosis associated with hepatitis B virus (HBV), and 8 patients (5 men and 3 women) aged 38 to 57 years old with cirrhosis of the liver on the background of combined HCV + HBV infection. The duration of the disease was 2–5 years. The presence of hepatitis B and C was established based on the detection of HBsAg and total anti-HCV antibodies respectively in the blood serum by ELISA.

The second group (II) included 65 people (39 women and 26 men) aged 24 to 81 years. Patients of this group were diagnosed with cirrhosis of the liver of unknown etiology, during which the persistence of herpes viruses—cytomegalovirus (CMV) and Epstein-Barr virus (EBV) was detected. The group did not include patients with lymphoproliferative diseases. The presence of herpes group viruses is detected when anti-infection antibodies to CMV and EBV are detected in the blood serum, in the absence of persistence of hepatitis A, B, C, and D viruses. The response of patients to infectious antigens was heterogeneous. We also detected in patients with liver cirrhosis and hepatosplenomegaly, autoantibodies to carotene-containing root crops were detected, which can be regarded as a trigger factor for this condition [65].

The third group (III) included 9 people (7 women and 2 men) aged 23 to 61 years. In patients, fatty hepatosis was diagnosed; the group was distinguished by frequent recurrent bleeding. In two patients of this group, the manifestation of bleeding began in childhood; this made it possible to suggest the presence of congenital storage diseases in this group patients. Further studies of the activity of lysosomal enzymes made it possible to confirm the presence of congenital genetically determined enzymopathy. Thus, the third group was characterized by hepatosplenomegaly against the background of a genetically determined deficiency of lysosomal enzymes (congenital enzymopathy).

In patients with hepatosplenomegaly, we used the following methods:

- ELISA – the presence of viral persistence: hepatitis HBV/HCV, CMV, EBV, *Helicobacter pylori*; the cytokine profile (IL-1β, IL-2, IL-6, IL-18, IFN-γ, TNF-α, IL-4, IL-10).

- Spectrophotometry – the level of various DAMP fractions (λ = 238 nm – oligopeptides, λ = 254 nm – peptides, λ = 260 nm – nucleotides, λ = 280 nm – aromatic amino acids), the content of ceruloplasmin and enzymes.

- Immunoturbidimetry – the concentration of C3 and C4 complement components.

- Light microscopy – the activity of oxygen-independent and oxygen-dependent phagocytosis; the level of lymphocytotoxicity in Terasaki test.

- Fluorescence microscopy – the presence of antiplatelet, antinuclear autoantibodies (ANA), and antineutrophil autoantibodies.

- Confocal microscopy – the reactive oxygen species (ROS) production.

- Flow cytometry – the state of adaptive immunity—the content of various subpopulations of T and B lymphocytes: B lymphocytes CD22+; T helpers CD3+CD4+; cytotoxic T lymphocytes CD3+CD8+/CD45+; early activation marker of the inflammatory process CD3+CD4+CD25+; regulatory T lymphocytes CD3+CD4+CD25+CD127-, costimulatory molecules CD3+CD4+CD28+, marker of T lymphocytes late activation CD3+HLA-DR+.

- Fluorimetry – the determination of enzymes β-glucocerebrosidal, tartrate-resistant acid phosphatase.

- Liquid chromatography – the content of amino acids.

3.5 The innate immunity factors in patients with hepatosplenomegaly

Some humoral (complement components) and cellular (activity of phagocytic neutrophils) factors that perform the main barrier function were studied.

In group I (HSM, hepatitis), the concentration of the C3 complement component was 117.0 ± 14.1 mg/dl and did not differ from the reference values (105.0 ± 7.1 mg/dl). There was a decrease in the activity of the C4 component (15.7 ± 3.11 mg/dl and reference values – 25.0 ± 1.12 mg/dl) due to its consumption in opsonization observations.

In group II (HSM, herpes viruses), a significant increase in the activity of the C3 component (up to 153.0 ± 6.3 mg/dL) was revealed, which led to the formation of a membrane attack complex, an additional tissue alteration factor.

The concentration of the C3 complement component in group III (enzymopathies) showed a slight increase (122.0 ± 8.4 mg/dl) against the background of the highest concentration of circulating immune complexes.

In group I was activation of the all stages of oxygen-independent phagocytosis (increased chemotaxis, adhesion, and absorptive capacity of neutrophils, as evidenced by significantly high values of the phagocytic index and phagocytic number) and pathological decrease in phagocyte endocytosis.

An increase in the phagocytic number by 42% indicated a high viral load or bacterial contamination, leading to an increase in the concentration of toxic DAMPs.

With intense adhesive and absorptive capacity of neutrophils, a pronounced pathological decrease (by 57%) in the phagocytosis completion index (0.71 ± 0.02 with a reference level of 1.21 ± 0.12) was revealed – endocytosis of antigens through lysosomal granzymes (**Table 1**).

A pronounced fourfold increase in the spontaneous level of NADPH-oxidase reactions of neutrophils was revealed in group I. Patients with HSM and hepatitis had a decrease in oxygen reserve, that is, an imbalance in the ratio of spontaneous and induced ROS production in NADPH-oxidase reactions of oxygen-dependent phagocytosis (**Table 1**).

To visualize the processing of antigen in neutrophils, we also used acridine orange dye, which made it possible to monitor the stages of DNA denaturation of the antigen (*Saccharomyces cerevisiae* cells), in the lysosomes of phagocytic neutrophils (**Figure 9A, B**).

In some patients of group II, neutrophil traps were detected (**Figure 9C**).

The number of neutrophil traps in patients of group II was the highest and amounted to 53.5%.

In group II (HSM, herpes viruses) was an excessive activation due to granzyme and mitochondrial enzyme complexes. And the magnitude of induced reactions was low, due to which there was a pathological ratio of spontaneous and induced reactions.

The stimulation index significantly decreased (**Table 1**).

Indicators	RV – reference values	Group I (HCV/HBV)	Group II (CMV/VEB)	Group III (congenital enzymopathy)
Oxygen-independent phagocytosis				
Phagocytic index,%	85.0 ± 5.1	98.8 ± 2.1*	91.0 ± 3.2	45.2 ± 2.7*
Phagocytic number	3.62 ± 0.2	5.1 ± 0.1*	4.77 ± 0.3*	2.1 ± 0.3*
Phagocytosis completion index	1.21 ± 0.12	0.71 ± 0.02*	0.95 ± 0.01*	0.8 ± 0.01*
Oxygen-dependent phagocytosis				
Spontaneous level of NADPH oxidase reactions (SP, %)	10.1 ± 1.1	44.48 ± 4.3*	29.23 ± 5.6*	25.0 ± 2.5*
Stimulated level of NADPH oxidase reactions (ST, %)	65.2 ± 3.2	66.69 ± 7.2	68.39 ± 5.9	71.5 ± 6.4
Stimulation index (SI=ST/SP)	6.5 ± 0.9	1.39 ± 0.4*	3.82 ± 0.6*	2.7 ± 0.3

*Note: * - the differences are reliable relative to the reference values, $p \leq 0.05$.*

Table 1.
Indicators of oxygen-independent and oxygen-dependent phagocytosis in patients with hepatosplenomegaly.

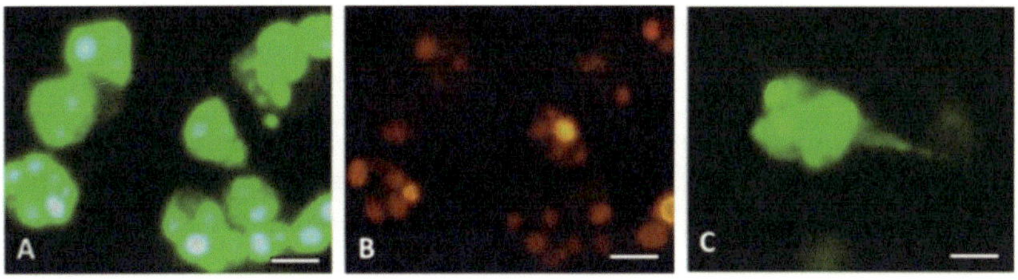

Figure 9.
Phagocytic activity of neutrophils: A – Native DNA, green color, λmax = 530 nm; B – Denatured DNA (incompleteness of the digestive function in oxygen-independent phagocytosis due to dysfunction of lysosomal enzymes, red color λmax = 640 nm); C – Formation of a neutrophil trap. The fluorescence color changed to red when the acridine orange dye was bound to denatured DNA of model antigen (S. cerevisiae). The intensity of red fluorescence characterized various functional stages of the activity of neutrophils lysosomal enzymes. The transition of double-stranded DNA to single-stranded DNA characterizes the intensive digestion of the antigen by neutrophil lysosomal enzymes, and undigested antigens retained the green luminescence of native DNA. Scale bar 10 μm. Fluorescence microscopy, magnification ×1000.

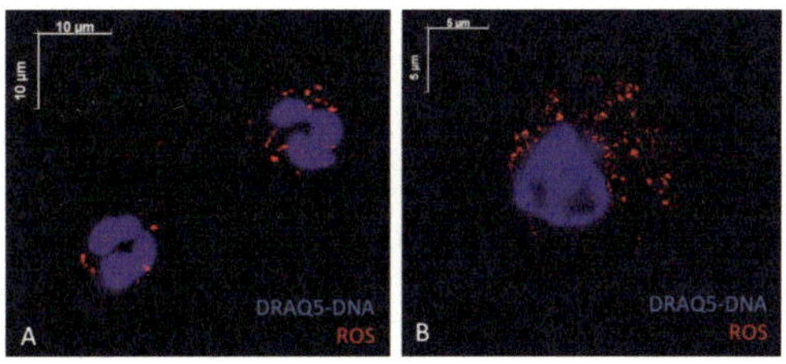

Figure 10.
Activation of neutrophils NADPH-reactions in oxygen-dependent phagocytosis due to mitochondrial enzyme complexes and massive formation of ROS, which contributed to the further free radical process. A – Intense ROS luminescence on phagocyte membranes during spontaneous unstimulated phagocytosis (scale bar 10 μm). B – A significant activation of the ROS formation after stimulation of NADPH oxidase reactions, an increase in the concentration of ROS on the membranes of the cytoplasmic structures of neutrophils (scale bar 5 μm). Nuclear DNA stained blue (DRAQ5 dye). Reactive oxygen species are stained red. Confocal microscopy.

Hyperactivation of the immune response in group II during inflammatory processes led to the development of oxidative stress. The production of reactive oxygen species (ROS) in neutrophils was five times higher than the reference level (measured in relative fluorescence units RFU = 3786.19), which caused increased cell apoptosis (**Figure 10**).

The production of ROS caused cell apoptosis, an increase in the activity of the neutrophil trap formation, and the activation of the gamma-glutamyl cycle enzymes involved in microsomal oxidation. The maximum increase (5.5 times) in the activity of gamma-glutamyltransferase indicated a violation of the gamma-glutamyl cycle antioxidant function, which is catalyzed by enzyme systems of the hepatocytes endoplasmic reticulum membranes with the participation of cytochrome p450.

Phagocytic reactions of neutrophils in group III (enzymopathy) differed significantly from the two previous groups in low ability to chemotaxis, adhesion, and endocytosis of antigens (**Table 1**). The failure of all stages of oxygen-independent phagocytosis indicated a defect in lysosomal enzymes, in particular beta-glucocerebrosidal, tartrate-resistant acid phosphatase, due to genetic deficiencies.

A threefold decrease in the catalytic activity of lysosomal enzymes is a diagnostic marker. A decrease in the activity of the enzymes lactate dehydrogenase and cholinesterase was also found.

3.6 Expression of lymphocyte differentiation clusters to enhance intercellular cooperation of immunocompetent cells

A chronic inflammatory response can be formed by DAMPs in the absence of acute infection or activation of endogenous PAMPs—cellular persisters [52, 66]. The cellular debris formed as a result of destruction, presented in the form of various endogenous cytotoxic DAMPs against the background of insufficiency of cellular and humoral factors of innate immunity, is also the cause of a change in the function of immunocompetent cells and a trigger factor for the autoimmune conditions development [67]. With ineffective reactions of innate immunity and the formation of an irreversible chronic inflammatory process in group I (hepatosplenomegaly, hepatitis), an increase in the expression of T lymphocytes late activation marker CD3+HLA-DR+ by 55% was revealed due to the long-term persistence of HBV and/or HCV viruses (**Figure 11**).

In group I, there was an increase in the concentration of profibrogenic pro-inflammatory cytokines IL-2 (8 times), IL-4 (6 times), IL-6 (18 times), and anti-inflammatory cytokine IL-10 (6 times), which initiate regeneration of destroyed hepatocytes by fibrotic type.

A twofold decrease in the expression of differentiation clusters of CD4+ T helpers and co-stimulating CD3+CD4+CD28+ cells led to a decrease in the activity of antibody-producing CD22+ B lymphocytes (by 13%) and impaired formation of specific clones of plasma cells.

In patients with a high content of the anti-inflammatory cytokine IL-10, the expression of regulatory Treg lymphocytes CD3+CD4+CD25+CD127- was reduced by 2.5 times due to the balance of pro-inflammatory cytokines.

In group I, a maximum twofold increase in the serum concentration of IgA was revealed, as a strong opsonizer and participant in the antigen-antibody-complement complex. This was probably due to the entry of large amounts of IgA contained in the intestinal mucosa through portosystemic anastomoses directly into the bloodstream during abdominal infection [68].

Group II (hepatosplenomegaly, herpes viruses) was the highest titer of antibodies to persistent VEB and CMV and a threefold increase in the number of CD22+ plasma B lymphocytes—antibody producers. Some patients had a high concentration of IgM and IgG, which characterizes the onset of inflammation and the active synthesis of virus-neutralizing antibodies and immune complexes.

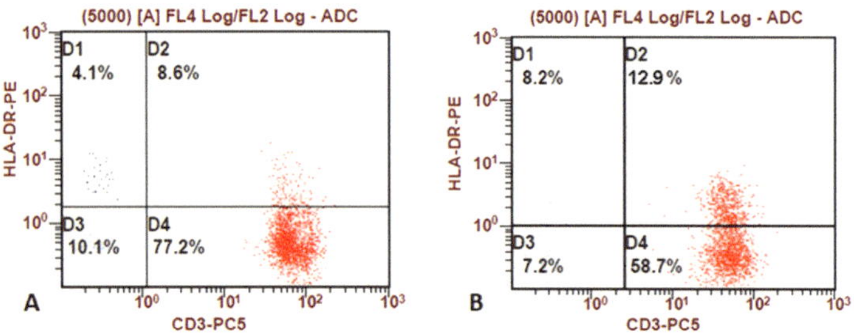

Figure 11.
Representative flow cytometry plots to determine the percentage of CD3+ T cells expressing HLA-DR. the number of cells with the CD3+HLA-DR+ phenotype is indicated by the D2 quadrant. As an example, individual values of the relative amount of the T lymphocytes late activation marker (CD3+HLA-DR+) are given: in a healthy donor (A), in a patient with hepatosplenomegaly on the background of HBV/HCV (B).

Some patients of group II had a compensatory increase in regulatory Treg cells CD3+CD4+CD25+CD127- in response to hyperactivation of pro-inflammatory cytokines.

From the revealed changes, it can be concluded that in group II patients with HSM against the background of herpes infection, humoral reactions prevailed and autoimmune processes were formed.

The high degree of intensity and severity of the inflammatory response in group II was characterized by another change in the profile of immune markers.

An increase in IL-1β (3 times), antiviral chemokine INF-γ (4 times), TNF-α (10 times)—the primary activators of acute inflammatory response —was revealed.

Some patients of group II had a multiple increase in IL-6 (18 times) and IL-18 (2 times). An increase in the synthesis of IL-6 leads to an increased entry of macrophages into the spleen. And an increase in IL-18 levels leads to the activation of macrophages that acquire a pro-inflammatory phenotype. Activated macrophages, together with CD8+ T lymphocytes infiltrate tissues, in particular the bone marrow and liver, and lead to cytopenia, liver dysfunction, and coagulopathies [69].

In group III, hepatosplenomegaly against the background of enzymopathy due to a defect in lysosomal enzymes was a decrease in primary inflammatory activators—IL-1β (2 times) and TNF-α (10 times). Anti-inflammatory IL-6 was increased by 20 times and characterized an increase in the intensity of inflammation against the background of bleeding.

In patients with hereditary enzymopathies, the highest iron content and a twofold increase in the vascular growth factor VEGF was revealed, which, in addition to stimulating angiogenesis, is a chemoattractant of Gaucher cells and an additional factor in their accumulation in the spleen and liver.

Also in group III, against the background of a normal content of serum immunoglobulins, a 1.5-fold increase in the subpopulation of CD22+ B lymphocytes was revealed.

3.7 The cytotoxic factors and DAMP fractions in patients with hepatosplenomegaly

In group I, an increase in the peptide fraction (λ = 254 nm) was revealed due to cytotoxic molecules of cell debris (DAMPs) and pathogen-associated molecular patterns (PAMPs), acting as autoimmunization inducers, as evidenced by the highest level of lymphocytotoxicity (in Terasaki test).

A twofold increase in the nucleotide fraction (λ = 260 nm) of average mass cytotoxic molecules was revealed due to the destruction of both the nuclear and mitochondrial genomes and their release into the intercellular space.

The concentration of ceruloplasmin, a plasma antioxidant, was reduced (by 40%) in patients with HSM on the background of hepatitis B and C (group I).

An increase in lactate and an adaptive fourfold increase in lactate dehydrogenase may also indicate in favor of mitochondrial dysfunction, which indicates a transition to glycolysis.

The increase in the fraction of aromatic amino acids (λ = 280 nm) is due to the high content of phenylalanine and tyrosine detected in the blood serum, which was detected in group II. In contrast to groups I and II, the oligopeptide fraction of average mass molecules (λ = 238 nm) in group III was increased.

The lipid profile of group III was characterized by an increased concentration of total cholesterol and a reduced concentration of high-density lipoproteins, which is characterized by a hereditary decrease in the lipoprotein lipase enzyme.

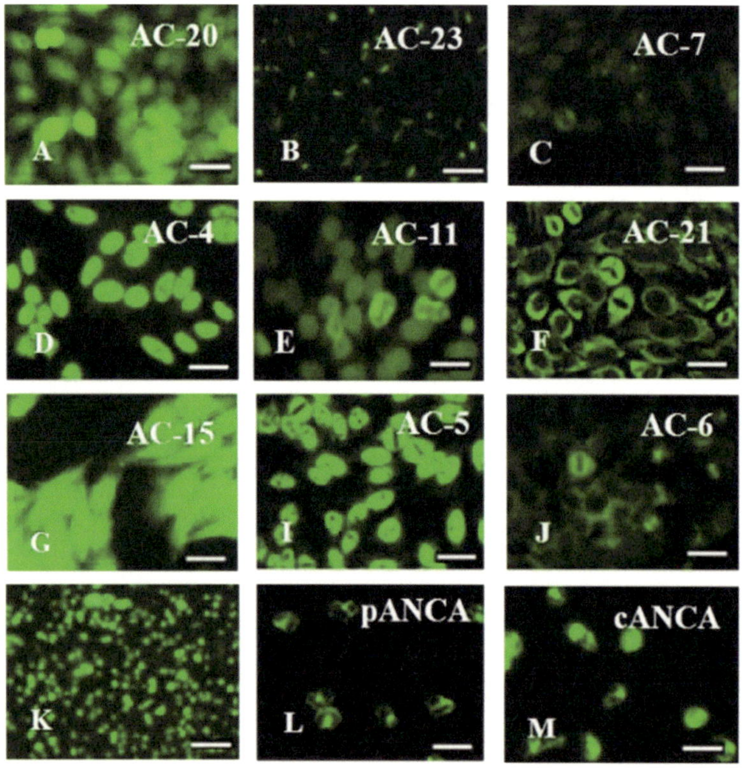

Figure 12.
Types of autoantibodies in patients with HSM of various etiologies. Antinuclear autoantibodies (ANA): A – To histidyl-tRNA synthetase; B – To filamentous structures; C – To the Cajal bodies; D – To SS-A/Ro, SS-B/La; E – To Lamin B; F – To mitochondria; G – To tropomyosin; I – To U1-RNP; J – To Sp-100, PML proteins; K – Antiplatelet antibodies; L – Perinuclear fluorescence type antineutrophil autoantibodies (pANCA); M – Cytoplasmic fluorescence type antineutrophil autoantibodies (cANCA). Fluorescent microscopy. Scale bar 20 μm. Codes AC (AC – Anti-cell pattern) in accordance with the international consensus on ANA patterns (ICAP) are presented. FITC staining of HEp-2 standard antigenic substrates after interaction with serum antibodies; magnification ×1000.

3.8 The repertoire of autoantibodies in hepatosplenomegaly

All examined patients with hepatosplenomegaly (HSM) had a large repertoire of autoantibodies: antiplatelet, antinuclear, and antineutrophil.

In group I, antinuclear autoantibodies (ANA) of 9 specificities with different frequency of occurrence were detected: to histidyl-tRNA synthetase in 12% (which is associated with antisynthetase syndrome); to dsDNA and histones in 5.9% (marker of high viral load); to centromeres in 5.8%; to Cajal bodies in 5.8% (containing small nuclear ribonucleoproteins involved in the processing of mRNA and histones, the restoration of telomeres, RNA splicing, and are also involved in reactions viral infection); to IMPDH2 (inosine monophosphate dehydrogenase 2) in 11.6%; to tropomyosin in 5.8%; to filamentous structures in 12%; to F-actin in 5.8% (controls and regulates the structural and functional features of the cytoskeleton) (**Figure 12**). Autoantibodies to Cajal bodies and tropomyosin were typical only for patients of group I.

The spectrum of autoimmune antibodies in group II (antiplatelet, antinuclear, antineutrophil, antimitochondrial, etc.) included 11 specificities.

Patients of group II had autoantibodies to platelets with the maximum frequency (in 95% of patients). The presence of autoantibodies to platelets in patients with HSM indicates their possible pathogenetic role in the occurrence of bleeding and thrombocytopenia. Thrombocytopenia found in group II due to the presence of autoantibodies to platelets, compensatory led to an increase in the production of plasma coagulation factors due to an increase in the concentration of fibrin and fibrinogen, which increase the risk of disseminated intravascular coagulation (DIC) condition.

In group II were detected antibodies to such antigens: dsDNA and histones (5.9%), centromeres (5.9%), histidyl-tRNA synthetase (5.9%), F-actin protein (5.9%), to soluble nuclear ribonucleoproteins SS-A/Ro and SS-B/La (18.2%), to protein MSA-2 (9.3%), to lamin B, PL7 (threonyl-tRNA synthetases) and PL12 (alanyl-tRNA synthetases) (9.1%), to mitochondria (17.6%) (**Figure 12**).

Since mitochondria are regulators of immunity, they control cell differentiation and induction. In addition, a significant contribution to the development of autoimmune reactions in HSM is made by mitochondrial dysfunction, which can be judged by the presence of antimitochondrial autoantibodies and dysfunction of mitochondrial complexes, leading to disruption of biochemical reactions cascades (accumulation of lactate, transition to glycolysis, disruption of cellular energy metabolism, Krebs cycle, cellular respiration, and β-oxidation).

Also in group II, the number of ANCA-positive patients was higher than in group I, and amounted to 85.7%. Among them, patients with the autoantibodies to the myeloperoxidase (pANCA – 71.4%) and to the proteinase 3 (cANCA – 14.3%) also prevailed (**Figure 12**).

Such a wide range of autoantibodies is the result of various factors of liver destruction and spleen tissues. Antibodies can have destructive processes; take part in cell killing, exerting a depressing effect on fibrogenic factors.

In group III (congenital enzymopathy), antinuclear antibodies ANA of two specificities were detected: to ribonucleoprotein U1-RNP (14.3%), involved in the initiation of pre-mRNA splicing, and Sp-100 and PML proteins (14.3%), which do not occur with viral etiology of HSM (**Figure 12**). Autoantibodies to PML proteins participate in transcription and apoptosis, in DNA repair and determining resistance to viruses. And the detected anti-PML autoantibodies prevent the inhibition of IL-6 secretion in this group.

3.9 Markers of autoimmune reactions in the choice of therapeutic targets for hepatosplenomegaly of various etiologies

Hepatosplenomegaly (HSM) is characterized by simultaneous enlargement of the spleen and liver in many hepatobiliary diseases. The dynamics of changes in HSM immune processes in response to various antigens occur with the activation and redistribution of cellular elements and changes in the functioning and reactivity primarily of the immunocompetent organ—the spleen [70, 71]. The method of choice for HSM against the background of portal hypertension and recurrent bleeding is splenectomy. But the effectiveness of splenectomy is not always appropriate, since a large number of specialized immune cells are removed from an important peripheral immunocompetent organ, which also performs the function of eliminating antigens.

A differential approach is needed to the choice of treatment tactics for patients in this category, taking into account reconstructive surgeries and targeted immunocorrection. In the Institute clinic, in patients with hepatosplenomegaly complicated by bleeding, the following types of operations are performed: devascularization of the esophageal cardia, sclerosis of the esophageal varices, splenorenal anastomoses in case of portal hypertension, embolization of the splenic artery, and in case of severe thrombocytopenia—splenectomy. Along with surgical treatment to eliminate the threat to the life of the patient due to bleeding, it is advisable to use transfusions of hematopoietic stem cells or cord blood [72] in group I. And in the II and III groups, it is advisable to use placental stem cell exometabolites in the form of exosomes to prevent active autoimmune processes.

The immunopathological markers found in patients indicate different mechanisms of HSM formation, depending on trigger factors and genetic predictors. Metabolic disorders in patients with HSM complicated by bleeding depend on the severity and duration of the stages of the inflammatory process, and the presence of an autoimmune component.

The identified immunological markers make it possible to substantiate a personalized diagnostic and treatment algorithm using specific antiviral antibodies, amino acids, transfusion of stem cells of various origin, anti-inflammatory cytokines and inhibitors of their receptors, and enzyme replacement therapy.

In group I patients (HSM against the background of HBV/HCV), the following was detected: activation of the secretion of profibrogenic pro-inflammatory cytokines IL-2, IL-4, IL-6; inhibition of the expression of the T lymphocytes early activation marker CD3+CD25+ and induction of the expression of the T lymphocytes late activation marker CD3+HLA-DR+; decrease in the C4 complement component due to its consumption as a cytolytic factor, followed by an increase in the peptide fraction of DAMP (λ = 254 nm); inhibition of phagocytic neutrophils endocytosis, which indicated the development of a chronic irreversible inflammatory reaction. These disorders contributed to the pronounced vascularization of the spleen tissues, which contributed to the development of the HSM syndrome. A high frequency of ANA autoantibodies occurrence, including those to Cajal bodies and tropomyosin, was revealed. In patients with HSM on the background of hepatitis viruses, an increase in the content of straight-chain amino acids and a multiple increase in the concentration of methionine were revealed, which indicates a violation of its metabolism to the end product, cysteine, which was significantly reduced.

For patients of group I, along with the correction of amino acid imbalance (disruption of the methionine cycle), it is advisable to use s-adenosyl methionine (SAMe), inosine, B vitamins (B6, B12), antiviral therapy with the use of interferons and other targeted drugs to support mitochondrial function, enzyme Q10, detoxification therapy (plasmapheresis), drugs to stimulate the adhesive function and endocytosis of phagocytes (composite drug Mix-Factor [73], stimulation of the synthesis of anti-inflammatory cytokines (recombinant IL-10, monoclonal antibodies to receptors of pro-inflammatory interleukins) (**Figure 13**).

In group II, patients in response to the persistence of CMV/EBV viruses, a multiple increase in the secretion of inducers of the inflammatory process first level—INF-γ, IL-1β, IL-18, TNF-α, and IL-6 was revealed, which reflected the severity of inflammatory reactions; induction of expression of T lymphocytes early activation marker CD3+CD4+CD25+; excessive stimulation of the ROS production and enhancement of NADPH reactions, which contributed to an increase in the frequency of neutrophil traps (NETs) formation; an increase in the cytolytic factor C3 complement component against the background of a multiple increase in the concentration of IL-1β and IL-18, it contributed to the intensive production of ROS and caspase-1-dependent cell pyroptosis. Patients in this group showed a high content of the cyclic amino acids fraction in the blood serum at λ = 280 nm.

And a different pattern of amino acid metabolism disorders was found, which was expressed in a significant increase in the titer of aromatic amino acids (phenylalanine, tyrosine), and a violation of the ornithine cycle. All patients of group II had antiplatelet antibodies, antineutrophil antibodies, and a wide range of antinuclear autoantibodies (ANA), including those to nuclear and mitochondrial nucleotides, causing mitochondrial dysfunction.

For patients of group II, it is advisable to use anti-inflammatory drugs (hormones, immunoglobulins, monoclonal antibodies, stimulants of innate immunity factors – Mix-Factor), cell membrane stabilizers (succinic acid, inosine, ascorbic acid, B vitamins), to reduce the autoimmune component–selenium preparations, therapy with amino acid preparations to correct disorders of the ornithine cycle, antioxidant therapy, stimulators of differentiation of the CD8+ killer subpopulation and CD16+ natural killers (**Figure 13**).

In group III, there was a lack of enzymes activity—β-glucocerebrosidase, tartrate-resistant acid phosphatase, and a pronounced decrease in lactate dehydrogenase and cholinesterase. Against the background of enzymopathy, all stages of oxygen-dependent and oxygen-independent phagocytosis were inhibited due to a defect in lysosomal enzymes; an increase in the concentration of inflammatory activators IL-1 and TNF-α was revealed. Pro-inflammatory IL-6 was elevated and characterized an increase in inflammation against the background of bleeding, and due to the development of an adaptive response, endothelial growth factor VEGF was increased. There was an increase in the DAMP oligopeptide fraction (λ = 238 nm), and a multiple increase in the serum iron content.

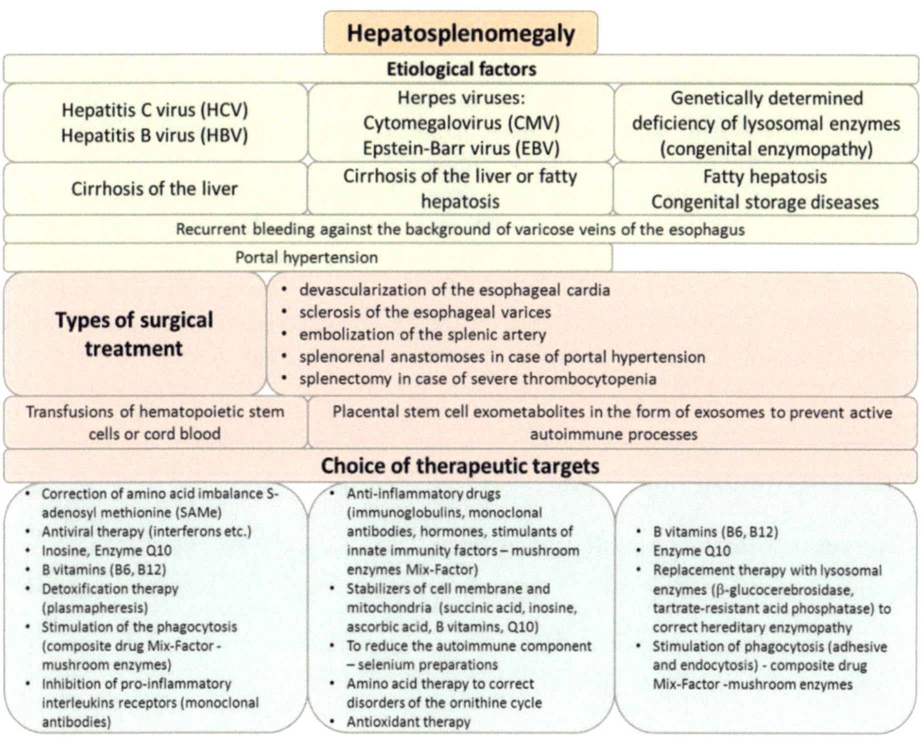

Figure 13.
The strategy of the treatments for patients with hepatosplenomegaly.

For patients of group III against the background of frequent recurrent bleeding—replacement therapy with lysosomal enzymes (beta-glucocerebrosidase, tartrate-resistant acid phosphatase) to correct hereditary enzymopathy, stimulation of phagocytosis (adhesive and digesting properties of phagocytes), it is advisable to use the composite drug Mix-Factor (**Figure 13**).

Thus, most patients with hepatosplenomegaly syndrome of varying severity, as a rule, require emergency surgical interventions. But it is necessary to take into account the presence of trigger factors and immunophysiological disorders in order to develop a comprehensive treatment and diagnostic algorithm, including targeted therapy of immune checkpoints, which will be the best option to prevent recurrence of bleeding in patients with hepatosplenomegaly.

4. Conclusions

Hepatosplenomegaly syndrome and myasthenia gravis are multifactorial diseases with an autoimmune component in pathogenesis. In these pathologies, immunocompetent organs are damaged. Myasthenia gravis is often accompanied by damage of the immunity central organ—the thymus, and structural and functional changes in the immunity peripheral organ—spleen, are associated with various diseases of the hepatobiliary system.

Myasthenia gravis and hepatosplenomegaly, which are often accompanied by portal vein hypertension and recurrent bleeding, are serious diseases. And their conservative treatment is not always effective and often these patients require emergency surgical care (thymectomy and splenectomy). Removal of immunocompetent organs may have negative consequences.

We have revealed trigger factors and predictors of autoimmune reactions in patients with various clinical phenotypes of myasthenia gravis and hepatosplenomegaly. The specific markers can be used to develop new treatment and diagnostic protocols and individual approaches to targeted therapy.

The identified specific markers characterize changes in the immune response and make it possible to choose individual treatment tactics and selectively apply surgical intervention in patients with thymus-independent myasthenia gravis, including certain HLA-DR polymorphism and a specific repertoire of autoantibodies; with splenomegaly— to correct autoimmune processes and excessive cellular proliferation in the spleen, and in the genetically determined orphan storage diseases to carry out enzyme replacement therapy.

Conflict of interest

The authors declare no conflict of interest.

Author details

Elena Klimova[1,2]*, Larisa Drozdova[1], Olena Lavinska[1,2], Sergey Sushkov[1] and Valery Boyko[1]

1 State Institution "Zaycev V. T. Institute of General and Urgent Surgery of National Academy of Medical Sciences of Ukraine", Kharkiv, Ukraine

2 V. N. Karazin National University, Kharkiv, Ukraine

*Address all correspondence to: klimovalena53@gmail.com

References

[1] Sharif K, Watad A, Coplan L, Lichtbroun B, Krosser A, Lichtbroun M, et al. The role of stress in the mosaic of autoimmunity: An overlooked association. Autoimmunity Reviews. 2018;**17**(10):967-983. DOI: 10.1016/j.autrev.2018.04.005

[2] Mathis D, Benoist C. Aire. Annual Review of Immunology. 2009;**27**:1,287-1,312. DOI: 10.1146/annurev.immunol.25.022106.141532

[3] Giraud M, Beaurain G, Yamamoto AM, Eymard B, Tranchant C, Gajdos P, et al. Linkage of HLA to myasthenia gravis and genetic heterogeneity depending on anti-titin antibodies. Neurology. 2001;**57**(9):1555-1560. DOI: 10.1212/wnl.57.9.1555

[4] Bach JF. The etiology of autoimmune diseases: The case of myasthenia gravis. Annals of the New York Academy of Sciences. 2012;**1274**:33-39. DOI: 10.1111/j.1749-6632.2012.06774.x

[5] Barreto R, Fagundes C, Guevara M, Solà E, Pereira G, Rodríguez E, et al. Type-1 hepatorenal syndrome associated with infections in cirrhosis: Natural history, outcome of kidney function, and survival. Hepatology. 2014;**59**(4):1505-1513. DOI: 10.1002/hep.26687

[6] Scarpino S, Di Napoli A, Stoppacciaro A, Antonelli M, Pilozzi E, Chiarle R, et al. Expression of autoimmune regulator gene (AIRE) and T regulatory cells in human thymomas. Clinical and Experimental Immunology. 2007;**149**(3):504-512. DOI: 10.1111/j.1365-2249.2007.03442.x

[7] Peterson P, Org T, Rebane A. Transcriptional regulation by AIRE: Molecular mechanisms of central tolerance. Nature Reviews. Immunology. 2008;**8**(12):948-957. DOI: 10.1038/nri2450

[8] Anderson MS, Venanzi ES, Chen Z, Berzins SP, Benoist C, Mathis D. The cellular mechanism of Aire control of T cell tolerance. Immunity. 2005;**23**(2):227-239. DOI: 10.1016/j.immuni.2005.07.005

[9] Xing Y, Hogquist KA. T-cell tolerance: Central and peripheral. Cold Spring Harbor Perspectives in Biology. 2012;**4**(6):a006957. DOI: 10.1101/cshperspect.a006957

[10] Lindstrom J, Anand R, Gerzanich V, Peng X, Wang F, Wells G. Structure and function of neuronal nicotinic acetylcholine receptors. Progress in Brain Research. 1996;**109**:125-137. DOI: 10.1016/s0079-6123(08)62094-4

[11] Conti-Fine BM, Milani M, Kaminski HJ. Myasthenia gravis: Past, present, and future. The Journal of Clinical Investigation. 2006;**116**(11):2843-2854. DOI: 10.1172/JCI29894

[12] Berrih-Aknin S, Frenkian-Cuvelier M, Eymard B. Diagnostic and clinical classification of autoimmune myasthenia gravis. Journal of Autoimmunity. 2014;**48-49**:143-148. DOI: 10.1016/j.jaut.2014.01.003

[13] Drachman DB. Myasthenia gravis. The New England Journal of Medicine. 1994;**330**:1797-1810. DOI: 10.1056/nejm199406233302507

[14] Vincent A. Unravelling the pathogenesis of myasthenia gravis. Nature Reviews. Immunology. 2002;**2**(10):797-804. DOI: 10.1038/nri916

[15] Verschuuren JJ, Huijbers MG, Plomp JJ, Niks EH, Molenaar PC, Martinez-Martinez P, et al. Pathophysiology of myasthenia gravis with antibodies to the acetylcholine receptor, muscle-specific kinase and low-density lipoprotein receptor-related protein 4. Autoimmunity Reviews. 2013;**12**(9):918-923. DOI: 10.1016/j.autrev.2013.03.001

[16] Stergiou C, Lazaridis K, Zouvelou V, Tzartos J, Mantegazza R, Antozzi C, et al. Titin antibodies in "seronegative" myasthenia gravis-a new role for an old antigen. Journal of Neuroimmunology. 2016;**292**:108-115. DOI: 10.1016/j.jneuroim.2016.01.018

[17] Gasperi C, Melms A, Schoser B, Zhang Y, Meltoranta J, Risson V, et al. Anti-agrin autoantibodies in myasthenia gravis. Neurology. 2014;**82**(22):1976-1983. DOI: 10.1212/WNL.0000000000000478

[18] Lazaridis K, Tzartos SJ. Autoantibody specificities in myasthenia gravis; implications for improved diagnostics and therapeutics. Frontiers in Immunology. 2020;**11**:212. DOI: 10.3389/fimmu.2020.00212

[19] Savino W, Dardenne M. Neuroendocrine control of thymus physiology. Endocrine Reviews. 2000;**21**(4):412-443. DOI: 10.1210/edrv.21.4.0402

[20] Armstrong SM, Schumann L. Myasthenia gravis: Diagnosis and treatment. Journal of the American Academy of Nurse Practitioners. 2003;**15**(2):72-78. DOI: 10.1111/j.1745-7599.2003.tb00354.x

[21] Melzer N, Ruck T, Fuhr P, Gold R, Hohlfeld R, Marx A, et al. Clinical features, pathogenesis, and treatment of myasthenia gravis: A supplement to the guidelines of the German neurological society. Journal of Neurology. 2016;**263**:1473-1494. DOI: 10.1007/s00415-016-8045-z

[22] Aydin Y, Ulas AB, Mutlu V, Colak A, Eroglu A. Thymectomy in myasthenia gravis. The Eurasian Journal of Medicine. 2017;**49**:48-52. DOI: 10.5152/eurasianjmed.2017.17009

[23] Farmakidis C., Pasnoor M., Dimachkie MM., Barohn R.J. Treatment of myasthenia gravis. Neurologic Clinics 2018; 36(2): 311-337. DOI:10.1016/j.ncl.2018.01.011

[24] Watanabe A, Watanabe T, Obama T, Mawatari T, Ohsava H, Ichmiya Y, et al. Prognostic factors for myasthenic crisis after transsternal thymectomy in patients with myasthenia gravis. Journal of thoracic and cardiovascular surgery. 2004;**127**(3):868-876. DOI: 10.1016/j.jtcvs.2003.07.036

[25] Bojko VV, Klimova EM, Kudrevich AN. Lechenie Miastenii s Uchetom Immunofiziologicheskih Fenotipov [Treatment of Myasthenia Gravis Taking into Account Immunophysiological Phenotypes]. Kharkov: Publishing House Sheinina E.V. 2008; p. 424

[26] Klimova EM, Lavinskaya EV, Minukhin DV, Syrovaya AO, Drozdova LA, Samoilova AP, et al. On forming central and peripheral markers of self-tolerance loss in diverse clinical Myasthenic phenotypes. Der Pharmacia Lettre. 2017;**9**(6):8-17. Available from: http://scholarsresearchlibrary.com/archive.html

[27] Sfriso P, Ghirardello A, Botsios C, Tonon M, Zen M, Bassi N, et al. Infections and autoimmunity: The multifaceted relationship. Journal of Leukocyte Biology. 2010;**87**(3):385-395. DOI: 10.1189/jlb.0709517

[28] Leopardi V, Chang Y-M, Pham A, Luo J, Garden OA. Systematic review of the potential implication of infectious agents in myasthenia gravis. Frontiers in Neurology. 2021;**12**:618021. DOI: 10.3389/fneur.2021.618021

[29] Eckl-Dorna J, Pree I, Reisinger J, Marth K, Chen K-W, Vrtala S, et al. The majority of allergen-specific IgE in the blood of allergic patients does not originate from blood-derived B cells or plasma cells. Clinical and Experimental Allergy. 2012;**42**(9):1347-1355. DOI: 10.1111/j.1365-2222.2012.04030.x

[30] Kumar H, Kawai T, Akira S. Pathogen recognition by the innate immune system. International Reviews of Immunology. 2011;**30**(1):16-34. DOI: 10.3109/08830185.2010.529976

[31] Skok MV, Koval LM, Lykhmus OY, Kalashnyk OM, Gergalova GL, Komisarenko SV. Nicotinic acetylcholine receptors: Specific antibodies and functions in humoral immunity Ukr. The Biochemical Journal. 2013;**85**(6):134-143. DOI: 10.15407/ubj85.06.134

[32] Hurst R, Rollema H, Bertrand D. Nicotinic acetylcholine receptors: From basic science to therapeutics. Pharmacology & Therapeutics. 2013;**137**(1):22-54. DOI: 10.1016/j.pharmthera.2012.08.012

[33] Bodis G, Toth V, Schwarting A. Role of human leukocyte antigens (HLA) in autoimmune diseases. Rheumatology and Therapy. 2018;**5**:5-20. DOI: 10.1007/s40744-018-0100-z

[34] Choo SY. The HLA system: Genetics, immunology, clinical testing, and clinical implications. Yonsei Medical Journal. 2007;**48**(1):11-23. DOI: 10.3349/ymj.2007.48.1.11

[35] Gough SC, Simmonds MJ. The HLA region and autoimmune disease: Associations and mechanisms of action. Current Genomics. 2007;**8**(7):453-465. DOI: 10.2174/138920207783591690

[36] Colbert RA, Tran TM, Layh-Schmitt G. HLA-B27 misfolding and ankylosing spondylitis. Molecular Immunology. 2014;**57**(1):44-51. DOI: 10.1016/j.molimm.2013.07.013

[37] Giraud M, Vandiedonck C, Garchon HJ. Genetic factors in autoimmune myasthenia gravis. Annals of the New York Academy of Sciences. 2008;**1132**:180-192. DOI: 10.1196/annals.1405.027

[38] Franciotta D, Cuccia M, Dondi E, Piccolo G, Cosi V. Polymorphic markers in MHC class II/III region: A study on Italian patients with myasthenia gravis. Journal of the Neurological Sciences. 2001;**190**(1-2):11-16. DOI: 10.1016/s0022-510x(01)00573-1

[39] Baecher-Allan C, Hafler DA. Suppressor T cells in human diseases. The Journal of Experimental Medicine. 2004;**200**(3):273-276. DOI: 10.1084/jem.20040812

[40] Kumar P, Saini S, Khan S, Surendra Lele S, Prabhakar BS. Restoring self-tolerance in autoimmune diseases by enhancing regulatory T-cells. Cellular Immunology. 2019;**339**:41-49. DOI: 10.1016/j.cellimm.2018.09.008

[41] Comacchio GM, Marulli G, Mammana M, Natale G, Schiavon M, Rea F. Surgical decision making: Thymoma and myasthenia gravis. Thoracic Surgery Clinics. 2019;**29**(2):203-213. DOI: 10.1016/j.thorsurg.2018.12.007

[42] Klimova EM, Minuchin DV, Drozdova LA, Lavinskaya EV, Kordon TI, Kalashnykova YV. Features of self-tolerance loss in patients with different

clinical phenotypes of myasthenia. Regulatory Mechanisms in Biosystems. 2018;**9**(4):561-567. DOI: 10.15421/021884

[43] Klimova EM, Drozdova LA, Lavinskaya EV, Minukhin DV, Kudrevych IO, Kudrevych OM. Genomic and epigenomic predictors for various clinical phenotypes of myasthenia gravis. Wiadomości Lekarskie. 2021;**LXXIV**(3):1. DOI: 10.36740/WLek202103117

[44] Bronte V, Pittet MJ. The spleen in local and systemic regulation of immunity. Immunity. 2013;**39**(5):806-818. DOI: 10.1016/j.immuni.2013.10.010

[45] Mihm S. Danger-associated molecular patterns (DAMPs): Molecular triggers for sterile inflammation in the liver. International Journal of Molecular Sciences. 2018;**19**(10):3104. DOI: 10.3390/ijms19103104

[46] Chentoufi AA, Serov YA, Alazmi M, Baba K. Immune components of liver damage associated with connective tissue diseases. Journal of Clinical and Translational Hepatology. 2014;**2**(1):37-44. DOI: 10.14218/JCTH.2014.00001

[47] Mogensen TH. Pathogen recognition and inflammatory signaling in innate immune defenses. Clinical Microbiology Reviews. 2009;**22**(2):240-273. DOI: 10.1128/CMR.00046-08

[48] Wu MY, Kao WY, Chan CY, Yiang GT, Liao WT, Chen CS. Spontaneous splenic rupture as a rare initial presentation in an acute lymphoblastic Leukemia patient. Diagnostics (Basel). 2019;**9**(4):152. DOI: 10.3390/diagnostics9040152

[49] Wong JL, Arango-Viana JC, Squires T. Heart, liver and spleen pathology in chronic alcohol and drug users. Journal of Forensic and Legal Medicine. 2008;**15**(3):141-147. DOI: 10.1016/j.jflm.2007.07.011

[50] Torimura T. Spleen and liver. The Liver in Systemic Diseases. 2016;**3**:35-50. DOI: 10.1007/978-4-431-55790-6_3

[51] Klimova EM, Bozhkov AI, Lavinska OV, Drozdova LA, Kurhuzova NI. Low molecular weight cytotoxic components (DAMPs) form the post-COVID-19 syndrome. Immunobiology. 2023;**228**(1):152316. DOI: 10.1016/j.imbio.2022.152316

[52] Vanderlugt CL, Miller SD. Epitope spreading in immune-mediated diseases: Implications for immunotherapy. Nature Reviews. Immunology. 2002;**2**(2):85-95. DOI: 10.1038/nri724

[53] Martinecz A, zur Wiesch PA. Estimating treatment prolongation for persistent infections. Pathogens and Disease. 2018;**76, 6**:fty065. DOI: 10.1093/femspd/fty065

[54] Koehli S, Naeher D, Galati-Fournier V, Zehn D, Palmer E. Optimal T-cell receptor affinity for inducing autoimmunity. Proceedings of the National Academy of Sciences USA. 2014;**111**:17248-17253. DOI: 10.1073/pnas.1402724111

[55] Mahanty S, Prigent A, Garraud O. Immunogenicity of infectious pathogens and vaccine antigens. BMC Immunology. 2015;**16**:31. DOI: 10.1186/s12865-015-0095-y

[56] Wucherpfennig KW. Mechanisms for the induction of autoimmunity by infectious agents. The Journal of Clinical Investigation. 2001;**108**(8):1097-1104. DOI: 10.1172/JCI14235

[57] Ercolini AM, Miller SD. The role of infections in autoimmune disease. Clinical and Experimental

Immunology. 2009;**155**(1):1-15. DOI: 10.1111/j.1365-2249.2008.03834.x

[58] Lv Y, Lau WY, Li Y, Deng J, Han X, Gong X, et al. Hypersplenism: History and current status. Experimental and Therapeutic Medicine. 2016;**12**(4):2377-2382. DOI: 10.3892/etm.2016.3683

[59] Lewis SM, Williams A, Eisenbarth SC. Structure and function of the immune system in the spleen. Science Immunology. 2019;**4**(33):eaau6085. DOI: 10.1126/sciimmunol.aau6085

[60] Zheng M, Tian Z. Liver-mediated adaptive immune tolerance. Frontiers in Immunology. 2019;**10**:2525. DOI: 10.3389/fimmu.2019.02525

[61] Dhar D, Baglieri J, Kisseleva T, Brenner DA. Mechanisms of liver fibrosis and its role in liver cancer. Experimental Biology and Medicine (Maywood, N.J.). 2020;**245**(2):96-108. DOI: 10.1177/1535370219898141

[62] Bozhkov AI, Novikova AV, Klimova EM, Ionov IA, Akzhyhitov RA, Kurhuzova NI, et al. Vitamin a reduces the mortality of animals with induced liver fibrosis by providing a multi-level body Defense system. Journal of Clinical and Experimental Hepatology. 2023;**13**(1):48-63. DOI: 10.1016/j.jceh.2022.09.006

[63] Bennett H, Troutman TD, Sakai M, Glass CK. Epigenetic regulation of Kupffer cell function in health and disease. Frontiers in Immunology. 2021;**11**:609618. DOI: 10.3389/fimmu.2020.609618

[64] Klimova EM, Drozdova LA, Lavinska OV, Bychenko EA, Kot YH, Kordon TI. Hepatosplenomegaly in liver cirrhosis is caused by reactive oxygen species formation, an increase in apoptosis and autophagy, and pronounced autoimmune reactions. Regulatory Mechanisms in Biosystems. 2021;**12**(3):408-418. DOI: 10.15421/022156

[65] Klimova EM, Kalashnikova YV, Merezhko OS, Kordon TI. Individual correction of the treatment of patients with hepatosplenomegaly syndrome, taking into account the parameters of lipid and protein metabolism. Kharkiv Surgical School. 2020;**5-6**:14-21. DOI: 10.37699/2308-7005.5-6.2020.03

[66] Chen L, Deng H, Cui H, Fang J, Zuo Z, Deng J, et al. Inflammatory responses and inflammation-associated diseases in organs. Oncotarget. 2017;**9**(6):7204-7218. DOI: 10.18632/oncotarget.23208

[67] Roh JS, Sohn DH. Damage-associated molecular patterns in inflammatory diseases. Immune Network. 2018;**18**(4):e27. DOI: 10.4110/in.2018.18.e27

[68] Klimova OM, Kordon TI, Sushkov SV, Drozdova LA, Lavinska OV, Merezhko OS, et al. Features of the immunoreactivity T and B lymphocytes subpopulations and cytokine imbalance in patients with hepatosplenomegaly of different etiology. Pathologia. 2021;**18**(2):174-182. DOI: 10.14739/2310-1237.2021.2.229454

[69] Grant S, Schulert A, Grom A. Macrophage activation syndrome and cytokine directed therapies. Best Practice & Research. Clinical Rheumatology. 2014;**28**(2):277-292. DOI: 10.1016/j.berh.2014.03.002

[70] Prasad AS, Halsted JA, Nadimi M. Syndrome of iron deficiency anemia, hepatosplenomegaly, hypogonadism, dwarfism and geophagia. The American Journal of Medicine. 1961;**31**:532-546. DOI: 10.1016/0002-9343(61)90137-1

[71] Liu P, Li P, He W, Zhao LQ. Liver and spleen volume variations in patients with hepatic fibrosis. World Journal of Gastroenterology. 2009;**15**(26):3298-3302. DOI: 10.3748/wjg.15.3298

[72] Boiko VV, Klymova OM, Vasylovska SV, Sushkov SV, Kordon TI, Shakina LO. Method for treatment of patients with the hepatocirrhosis and prevention of its complications. Pat. No. 37688, A61K 45/00. Published 10.12.2008, Bulletin No. 23. 2008:1-6

[73] Bozhkov A, Ivanov I, Klimova E, Kurguzova N, Bozhkov A, Goltvyanskiy A, et al. "Mix-factor" is involved in the regulation of the organism's redox systems in the late stages of ontogenesis and affects the lifespan of animals. Ageing and Longevity. 2021;**2**(2):24-36. DOI: 10.47855/jal9020-2021-2-4

Chapter 4

Mortality Causes of Autoimmune Rheumatic Diseases

Maynor Herrera-Méndez

Abstract

Autoimmune Rheumatic Diseases (ARDs) are chronic multisystemic diseases that have a low prevalence (estimated to range from 4 to 5% of the general population), and the impact on mortality in ARDs is lower (mortality reported in ARDs is 0.3 to 2.1) in general statistics worldwide compared to other diseases with higher prevalence such as arterial hypertension (HBP) or diabetes mellitus (DM). The objective of this review is to update the concepts regarding mortality associated with ARD, and the most relevant studies and review were included. The causes of mortality among ARDs vary widely between geographic areas and cannot be generalized, although the most important frequency reported is in rheumatoid arthritis (RA), systemic lupus erythematosus (SLE) and scleroderma (SSc). It has recently been reported that measuring the standardized mortality rate (SMR) identifies the inflammatory diseases with increased risk: 4.80 in systemic vasculitis (SV), 2.9 in SLE, and 1.44 in RA. The causes of death are regularly associated with acute events (infections and respiratory and cardiovascular diseases) and less frequent related to the disease severity. Other reported associated factors have been age, duration, type of presentation of the disease, and socioeconomic status. We found that the variation between the main reported causes is little; significantly higher mortality (five times more) has been found in the regional analysis in Latin America compared to that in Europe. The most important factor in the last decades is the habitual use of drugs that increase the risk of immunosuppression and infection.

Keywords: autoimmune rheumatic diseases, systemic vasculitis, systemic lupus erythematosus, rheumatoid arthritis, standardized mortality ratio

1. Introduction

Autoimmune rheumatic diseases have a low prevalence of associated mortality (0.3 to 2.1) [1]. When the mortality of ARDs is compared with more prevalent diseases (DM and BHP), the statistical impact is lower worldwide, and consequently, the study of its causes has been limited.

The objective of this review is to update the concepts on mortality associated with ARD, and we searched for studies of the last 50 years in the main databases (Pubmed, Cochrane, Google academic, and Scopus) using the words autoimmune disease, rheumatic disease, and mortality in autoimmune disease and then looking for causes of mortality in VS, SLE, and RA.

IntechOpen

The information analyzed comes from databases of better organized institutions and complemented with the analysis of studies that describe in detail the causes of mortality in the different latitudes; sixty-five reports (cases, observational studies, and database analysis) of mortality and rheumatic disease were reviewed, including at the end 25 that contain the most important information.

Recently was informed that measure the standardized mortality ratio risk identified at population in risk. In general terms, the group of rheumatic diseases has a risk of 2.03 (95% CI: 1.79–2.29) and has been reported particularly for those considered as inflammatory. The highest risk reported was 4.80 in systemic vasculitis, followed by 2.9 in systemic lupus erythematosus and 1.44 in rheumatoid arthritis [2].

Some studies also report that patients with diseases such as Myositis (MI), SSc, and Sjogren's syndrome (SS) may have a significant risk, which is not yet considered among the most important because its prevalence is lower.

The causes of death are regularly associated with acute events, infections, cardiovascular and lung diseases, and a lower probability with the clinical spectrum of the disease.

Other related factors reported are age and duration of the disease, the severity of presentation, and the adverse effects relating to the treatment administered [3–5]. The comorbidities, specialty cardiovascular, metabolic, and respiratory are the most important [6–8].

Most recently, use of novelty pharmacies (monoclonal antibodies, Jak inhibitors) in combination with glucocorticoids and immunosuppressive drugs has been proposed as the factor that increases the risk [9–12]. However, it should be noted that thanks to this therapeutic innovation, ARD patients have improved their quality and life expectancy.

2. Development of mortality study in ARD

2.1 General features

The notion of autoimmune diseases in humans' dates to the beginning of the 20th century, and currently, more than 40 human diseases have been described that could have this name.

The first widely described autoimmune disease with underlying pathophysiological mechanisms was Hemolytic Anemia, described in 1925 by Lederle [13]. However, autoimmune diseases were not officially recognized as such until the 1940s–50s, and until then, the reports on mortality in these diseases were scarce. The first congress on these diseases was held in 1965.

In this line of time (**Figure 1**), the main events related to autoimmune diseases are identified.

2.2 Background

The study of rheumatic diseases focused on morbidity, loss of function, instability caused by joint damage, and reduced quality of life. Nonetheless, in 1955, it was estimated that the 5-year survival in patients with SLE, vasculitis, and polymyositis was only 5%, and it was considered part of the "natural history" of the disease; it was considered that the systemic inflammatory process and the progression of disease were the cause of death [14].

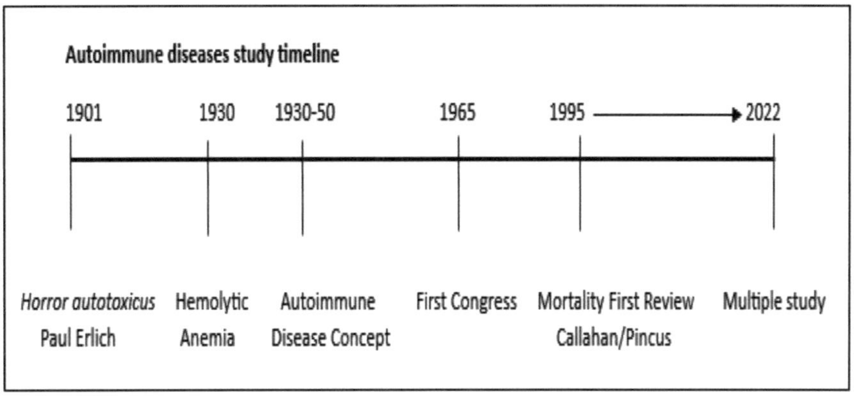

Figure 1.
Line of time.

As early as 1953, Cobb et al. described the course of death in 130 patients with rheumatoid arthritis who were followed for nine years. The first cause of death reported in 25% was infection, 24% heart disease and 13% various forms of nephropathy [15]; besides, in similar study, Mitchell reported a decrease in 5–15 years life expectancy in this patient [16].

In 1976, Urowitz and his collaborators suggested bimodality as the cause of death in SLE: 1. Early death with an active disease that requires high doses of glucocorticoids is regularly associated with infections and 2. A late death in an inactive disease, which has required many years of glucocorticoid intake and whose outcome is heart disease [17].

2.3 Current development in mortality trends

Due to the wide variation in mortality in rheumatic diseases, it has been necessary to develop precise and weighted analyses that calculate the risk; one of them is the SMR. This is obtained by calculating the relationship between the deaths observed in a cohort and those expected in a group of the same size from the general population (in the same area and standardized by age and sex).

Toledano et al. measured the SMR in rheumatic diseases and performed a meta-analysis in 2012, finding 32 studies that were analyzed (16 in RA, 7 in SC, 5 in SLE, and 2 in Vasculitis). They reported that the highest risk is in inflammatory diseases, vasculitis 4.8, SLE 2.9, and RA 1.4, and reported that the leading cause of mortality is cardiovascular diseases, followed by pulmonary, renal, and infectious diseases [2]. In ARDs with an inflammatory component, SMR 2.03 is higher and becomes evident when compared with that of fibromyalgia, an entity without an inflammatory burden, with 0.49 [18].

Recently, in 2020, Scherlinger and collaborators have carried out a review of the mortality of rheumatic diseases between 2001 and 2014; the six main diseases, SLE, SSC, MI, SS, Vasculitis, and MCTD (mixed connective tissue disease), reported according to the World Health Organization were included. The number of deaths per million inhabitants was estimated using the ASMR (aged-standardized mortality rate), with the most important data being SLE 2.68 and SSc 1.48. The following were reported during 2014 (reports from 35 to 85 countries): 6418 deaths in SLE, 4287 in SSc, 1313 in MI, 438 in SS, 235 in MCTD, and 1350 in Vasculitis [19].

It is found that the ASMR is up to five times higher in the countries of Latin America compared to the in the countries of Europe, not finding this relationship with countries of other continents [19]. This could be related to inequity in the provision of medical care and the quality of health services in each of the countries that consistently report mortality.

3. Autoimmune predisposition

3.1 Background

ARDs are a heterogeneous group of diseases, characterized by an immune dysregulation resulting in inflammation and multi-organ involvements that can conditioned the died.

The immune dysregulation involves tissues, cells, and molecules that usually participated in immune response, especially against infectious agents [20].

Usually factors involved in this dysregulation are several: Ambiental, genetic, infectious diseases, and most recent changes in the microbiome and hygienic hypothesis.

Because of this initial stimulus, the immune response has become unbalanced, and our own tissues become the target of action, named *horror autotoxicus* for Paul Erlich in 1901 [20].

This imbalance is reflected in the different pathways that participate in the immune response, which react to the presence of an "autoantigen" that is not recognized as their own (loss of self-tolerance), because the peptide sequences are similar and can be confused with those of foreign agents.

3.2 Hypothesis and ARD development

In recent years, different hypotheses have been accepted as triggers for an autoimmune disease; the most important are [21]: Exposure of cryptic antigens, overexpression of MHC (Major Histocompatibility Complex) and costimulatory molecules, neoantigen (microorganism + self-antigen), super antigen (polyclonal activation of T lymphocytes), and molecular mimicry.

Initially, the autoantigen is caught for antigen presenting cells (APC) and presented to the T cells in the thymus, in response the most autoreactive T cells that undergo apoptosis, but a small percentage of them enter the general circulation and escape the usual controls: clonal anergy (in peripheral lymphoid tissue), phenomenon of suppression by Treg cells and immunological ignorance (whose mechanisms are still unknown).

These reactive T cells are responsible for activating B cells that produce and release specific antibodies and proinflammatory cytokines, which in turn are responsible for amplifying inflammation and triggering the phenomena of tissue destruction and the systemic manifestations of autoimmune diseases, which can be perpetuated and cause death of the patient [21].

Figure 2 illustrates the process of generalized inflammation, with the possible triggers for an ARD and the factors that contribute to death as the outcome. Timely therapeutic intervention (pharmacological or non-pharmacological) can change the outcome.

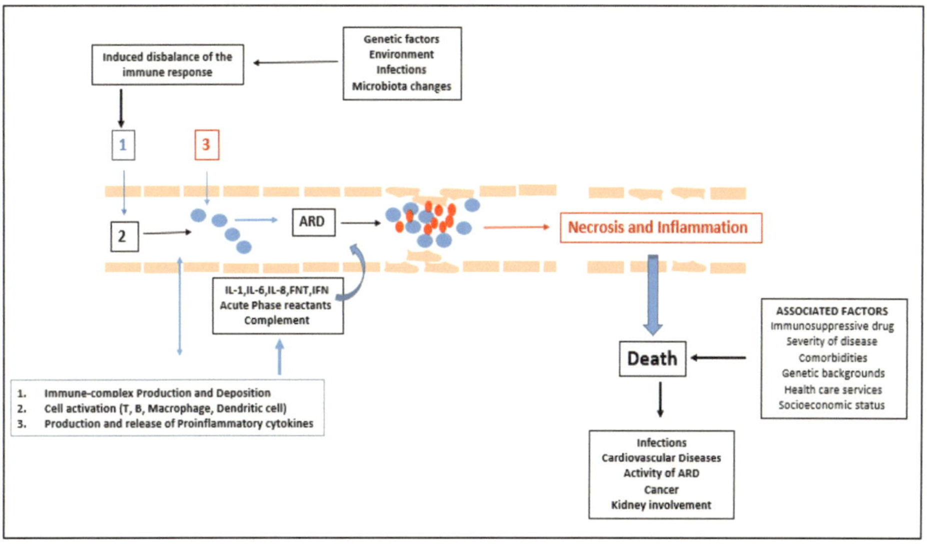

Figure 2.
ARD development.

4. Comorbidities associated with mortality in ARD

4.1 Background and reports

In recent years, data collection through population-based studies has increased; it is the most widely used method for analyzing the prevalence of comorbidities.

However, it is pertinent in the analysis to establish that it requires considerable resources and the self-filling of documents by the patients, which implies the probability of making errors in the identification of the main pathologies, especially in the case of ARDs, which are diseases with great clinical and complex heterogeneity.

The report of various studies has assessed the co-occurrence of ARD with other diseases at the time of death, regularly using death certificate data, among the most frequent is include to cardiovascular diseases, pulmonary disorders, coagulation and hemorrhagic disorders, and renal failure.

We have reported in our center the mortality-associated comorbidities in ARD; those of the highest prevalence were HBP at 38.9% and DM type II at 11.3%. Specifically, in SLE, 50% reported HBP, 8.7% antiphospholipid syndrome (APS) associated with thrombosis, and 6.5% chronic kidney disease (CKD). In RA, the main association was HBP in 26.9% and DM-II in 23% of cases. In 24.3%, no comorbidity was reported [22].

These data are like those reported by another investigators: Panoulas et al. and Petri et al. reported in RA and SLE the double the prevalence of HBP in comparison with the general population [6, 7].

Sabio et al. reported HBP in 40% of patients with SLE compared with the 11% of controls of the same age [8].

Other authors also include minor comorbidities, musculoskeletal disease, genitourinary system, blood diseases, and diseases of the skin and subcutaneous tissue, and confirm the classic cause, cardiovascular diseases (55.5%), followed by diseases of the respiratory system (35.9%), endocrine and metabolic disorders (21.6%), and neoplasms (20.9%) [23].

4.2 Analysis of identified risks

The vascular compromise suggested the close relationship between the constant inflammatory states that affect the blood vessels, especially in the heart, kidney, and the central and peripheral nervous system.

The importance of therapeutic intervention is vital; however, it is not free of complications. This could explain the bimodal presentation of mortality reported by Urowitz [17].

The use of corticosteroids, immunosuppressants such as cyclophosphamide, and, recently, monoclonal antibodies decreases the risk of progression of the disease by controlling inflammation but increases the risk of infection.

In the case of metabolic diseases, especially DM type II could be secondary at use of glucocorticoids and lifestyle patterns no modified that increase the risk of death secondary to immunosuppression and vascular diseases associated. The use of concomitant drugs to control glucose levels and blood pressure continuously contributes to a good control of the disease and a better outcome.

5. Therapeutics and ARD mortality

Survival of patients with ARD in the last 5 decades has improved significantly due to the use of medications such as glucocorticoids, immunosuppressants, monoclonal antibodies, and concomitant drugs (antihypertensive agents, antibiotics, etc.).

However, for the extended use of glucocorticoids, there has also been an increase in the risk of developing infections. Saag et al. reported an 8 times increased risk (OR) compared to those who do not use them [9].

Petri et al. reported a higher risk of infection when comparing patients with SLE with and without hospitalization, with doses of prednisone higher than 10 mg/day [7], and Listing et al. in RA found that doses of glucocorticoids above 5 mg were associated with an increase in mortality [10].

In general terms, an increased risk of death has not been demonstrated with the use of immunosuppressants; two authors, Bultink and Listing, reported a lower risk of mortality (not statistically significant) in patients with SLE intake any immunosuppressant drugs [10, 11], and Mok et al. highlight that the use of immunosuppressants was not associated with increased survival in patients with SLE; however, the risk of infections increases considerably [12].

6. Mortality around the world

In recent years, the number of studies on the causes of mortality in ARDs has increased, although the methodologies used are diverse; the results of most studies show infections as the main cause, followed by cardiovascular and pulmonary diseases.

Some studies have also described disease activity as the cause of death, and it stands out that at least two of them report the cause of death as missing or unknown.

Recently, in a population study in Greece, Bournia et al. have described that mortality in rheumatic diseases occurs more frequently compared to the general population, preferably in young patients and the prevalence is higher in the main inflammatory diseases (SLE, SV and SSC) [24].

Author/Country	Year study/ patients number	Mortality causes (%)	Reference/comments
Mok et al./Hong Kong	1999–2008/2486	Infections (28%) CV complications (18%) Cancer (16%) Disease activity (7%) Renal failure (6%) Pulmonary causes (6%) GI/Hepatic complications (4%) Accidents, injury, or poisoning (including suicide) (0.7%) Missing (9%)	[5]
Toledano et al./ Spain	2012	SMR high risk Infections 11.3 CV 3 Pulmonary causes 2.33	[2] Meta-analysis
Garen et al./ Norwegian	1999–2015/279	CV (27%) SV (28%) Cancer (CTD 25%-SV 27%), Pulmonary causes (CTD 20%-SV10%) Infections (CTD 9%-SV 16%).	[25] Ten-year follow
Mitratza et al./ Netherlands	2013–2017/ 3335	CV (55.5%) Respiratory causes (35.9%) Endocrine and metabolic disorders (21.6%) Cancer (20.9%) Infections (16%) Musculoskeletal system 3.38 Genitourinary system 2.73 Influenza 2.71 Blood diseases 2.02 Skin and subcutaneous tissue diseases 1.95 Infectious diseases 1.85	[23]
Dadoniene J et al./ Lithuanian	2013–2019/950	CV (47%) Cancer (23%) Respiratory causes (6%) Musculoskeletal system (5%) Other causes (16%)	[26] Patients with ARD have a higher risk of mortality and lower life expectancy
Leonardo H et al./ Guatemala	2009–2019/185	Infections (56%) Activity Disease (16%) CV (8%) Other (7%) Unknown (12%)	[22]

CV, cardiovascular; SMR, standardized mortality ratio; CTD, Connective Tissue Disease; SV, Systemic vasculitis.

Table 1.
Main cause of mortality around the world.

It is possible that factors such as the quality of care provided by health services and the socioeconomic conditions of the patients are not correctly recorded, and for now, it is not possible to establish a direct relationship with these factors that are mentioned anecdotally as contributors to the mortality of the ARDs.

The consensus is that effective therapeutic modalities such as treat-to-target and effective control of comorbidities improve survival and, with experience obtained with this methodology in RA and EA during the years 2015–2019, should be extended to all ARDs [24].

Table 1 summarizes the most important studies in recent years and identifies the main causes. Most agree in reporting that infections, CV and pulmonary complications, and disease activity are the leading causes of death.

It also allows you to view the comorbidities that are reported as a product of the same disease, associated with the disease or consequence of the therapeutic used, such as HBP, endocrine and metabolic diseases, kidney failure, liver complications, and cancer.

7. Conclusion

We found that the variation between the main reported causes is little; the results of most studies show infections as the main cause, followed by cardiovascular and pulmonary diseases.

The risk is largely different among various ARDs, due to diverse underlying pathogenetic mechanisms and the degree of vital organ involvement, as well as due to different therapeutic regimes used and different age of onset of each disease.

The higher mortality (five times more) that has been reported in Latin America compared to in Europe is significantly important. It could be related to the quality and inequity in the provision of health services; this analysis is beyond this review.

The most important factor in the last decades is the habitual use of drugs that increase the risk of immunosuppression and infection. It is common that the ARDs are characterized by increased morbidity and mortality, due to disease-specific factors and iatrogenic damage (e.g., drug-related side effects) and the associated comorbidity as cardiovascular disease, malignancy, and increased risk for infections.

The routine electronic or manual recording systems for death, admissions, and hospital discharge statistics provide only a partial picture of the prevalence of ARDs and could be the reason why these diseases have a low lethality and hospitalization frequency.

Conflict of interest

The author does not have conflict of interests to declare.

Funding

This research did not receive any specific funding from public sector, commercial sector, or not-for-profit agencies.

Author details

Maynor Herrera-Méndez
Internal Medicine Department, Rheumatology Unit - Roosevelt Hospital, Post Graduate School of San Carlos University of Guatemala, Guatemala

*Address all correspondence to: drherreram@gmail.com

References

[1] Thomas SL, Griffiths C, Smeeth L, Rooney C, Hall AJ. Burden of mortality associated with autoimmune diseases among females in the United Kingdom. American Journal of Public Health. 2010;**100**:2279-2287. Available from: https://ajph.aphapublications.org/doi/abs/10.2105/AJPH.2009.180273

[2] Toledano E, Candelas G, Rosales Z, Martínez C, León L, Abásolo L, et al. A meta-analysis of mortality in rheumatic diseases. Reumatología Clínica. 2012;**8**:334-341. DOI: 10.1016/j.reuma.2012.05.006

[3] Tselios K, Gladman D, Sheane B, Su J, Urowitz M. All-cause, cause-specific and age-specific standardized mortality ratios of patients with systemic lupus erythematosus in Ontario, Canada over 43 years (1971-2013). Annals of the Rheumatic Diseases. 2019;**78**:802-806. DOI: 10.1136/annrheumdis-2018-214802

[4] Martinez M, Quinteros C, Abud C. Hospitalizations and mortality in Mexican patients with systemic lupus erythematosus (SLE) or rheumatoid arthritis (RA). Annals of the Rheumatic Diseases. 2014;**73**(Suppl. 2):115. DOI: 10.1136/annrheumdis-2014-eular.4784

[5] Mok C, Kwok L, Ho L, Chan P, Yip S. Life expectancy, standardized mortality ratios, and causes of death in six rheumatic diseases in Hong Kong, China. Arthritis and Rheumatism. 2011;**63**:1182-1189. DOI: 10.1002/art.30277

[6] Panoulas V, Metsios G, Pace A, John H, Treharne G, Banks M, et al. Hypertension in rheumatoid arthritis. Rheumatology (Oxford, England). 2008;**47**:1286-1298. DOI: 10.1093/rheumatology/ken159

[7] Petri M, Mease P, Merrill J, Lahita R, Iannini M, Yocum D, et al. Effects of prasterone on disease activity and symptoms in women with active systemic lupus erythematosus. Arthritis and Rheumatism. 2004;**50**:2858-2868. DOI: 10.1002/art.20427

[8] Sabio J, Vargas-Hitos J, Navarrete-Navarrete N, Mediavilla J, Jiménez-Jáimez J, Díaz-Chamorro A, et al. Prevalence of and factors associated with hypertension in young and old women with systemic lupus erythematosus. The Journal of Rheumatology. 2011;**38**:1026-1032. DOI: 10.3899/jrheum.101132

[9] Saag KG, Koehneke R, Caldwell JR, Brasington R, Burmeister LF, Zimmerman B, et al. Low dose long-term corticosteroid therapy in rheumatoid arthritis: An analysis of serious adverse events. The American Journal of Medicine. 1994;**96**:115-123. DOI: 10.1016/0002-9343(94)90131-7

[10] Listing J, Kekow J, Mangere B. Mortality in rheumatoid arthritis: The impact of disease activity, treatment with glucocorticoids, TNF inhibitors and rituximab. Annals of the Rheumatic Diseases. 2015;**74**:415-421. DOI: 10.1136/annrheumdis-2013-204021

[11] Bultink I, de Vries F, van Vollenhoven R, Lalmohamed A. Mortality, causes of death and influence of medication use in patients with systemic lupus erythematosus vs matched controls. Rheumatology. 2020;**00**:1-10. DOI: 10.1093/rheumatology/keaa267

[12] Mok C, Tse S, Chan K. Effect of immunosuppressive therapies on survival of systemic lupus erythematosus:

A propensity score analysis of a longitudinal cohort. Lupus. 2017;**27**:722-727. DOI: 10.1177/0961203317739129

[13] Lederer M. Form of acute hemolytic anemia-probably of infectious origin. American Journal of Medical Sciences. 1925;**170**:500-510

[14] Callahan L, Pincus T. Mortality in the rheumatic diseases. Arthritis Care and Research. 1995;**8**:229-241. DOI: 10.1002/art.1790080406

[15] Cobb S, Anderson F, Bauer W. Length of life and cause of death in rheumatoid arthritis. The New England Journal of Medicine. 1953;**249**:553-556. DOI: 10.1056/nejm195310012491402

[16] Mitchell DM, Spitz PW, Young DY, Bloch DA, Mc-Shane DJ, Fries JF. Survival, prognosis, and causes of death in rheumatoid arthritis. Arthritis and Rheumatism. 1986;**29**:706-714. DOI: 10.1002/art.1780290602

[17] Urowitz M, Bookman A, Koehler GD, Smythe H, Ogryzlo M. The bimodal mortality pattern of systemic lupus erythematosus. The American Journal of Medicine. 1976;**60**:221-225. DOI: 10.1016/0002-343(76)90431-9

[18] Wolfe F, Hassett AL, Walitt B, Michaud K. Mortality in fibromyalgia: A study of 8,186 patients over thirty-five years. Arthritis Care & Research (Hoboken). 2011;**63**:94-101. DOI: 10.1002/acr.20460

[19] Scherlinger M, Mertz P, Sagez F, Meyer A, Felten R, et al. Worldwide trends in all-cause mortality of auto-immune systemic diseases between 2001 and 2014. Autoimmunity Reviews. 2020;**19**:102531. DOI: 10.1016/j.autrev.2020.102531

[20] Plotz PH. Autoimmunity: The history of an idea. Arthritis and Rheumatism. 2014;**66**:2915-2920. DOI: 10.1002/art.38796

[21] Pollard K, Hultman P, Kono D. Immunology and genetics of induced systemic autoimmunity. Autoimmunity Reviews. 2005;**4**:282-288. DOI: 10.1016/j.autrev.2004.12.005

[22] Leonardo H, Carrascosa M, Arreola R, Herrera-Méndez M. Causes of mortality associated with autoimmune rheumatic disease in a referral hospital. Reumatología Clínica. 2022;**18**:304-308. DOI: 10.1016/j.reuma.2021.02.010

[23] Mitratza M, Klijs B, Hak E, Kardaun J, Kunst A. Systemic autoimmune disease as a cause of death: Mortality burden and comorbidities. Rheumatology. 2021;**60**:1321-1330. DOI: 10.1093/rheumatology/keaa537

[24] Bournia V, Fragoulis G, Mitrou P, Mathioudakis K, Tsolakidis A, Konstantonis G, et al. All-cause mortality in systemic rheumatic diseases under treatment compared with the general population, 2015-2019. RMD Open. 2021;**7**:e001694. DOI: 10.1136/rmdopen-2021-001694

[25] Garen T, Lerang K, Hoffmann-Vold A, Andersson H, Midtvedt Q, Brunbor C, et al. Mortality and causes of death across the systemic connective tissue diseases and the primary systemic vasculitides. Rheumatology. 2019;**58**:313-320. DOI: 10.1093/rheumatology/key285

[26] Dadoniene J, Charukevic G, Jasionyte G, Staškuviene K, Miltiniene D. Mortality in inflammatory rheumatic diseases: Lithuanian National Registry Data and systematic review. International Journal of Environmental Research and Public Health. 2021;**18**:12338. DOI: 10.3390/ijerph182312338

Chapter 5

Etiology and Pathogenesis of Buerger's Disease

Ping Zheng and WanChao Wang

Abstract

This chapter delves into the multifaceted etiology of Buerger's disease, also known as thromboangiitis obliterans (TAO), exploring a spectrum of factors contributing to its onset and the initiation of vascular inflammation. We comprehensively summarize our research findings regarding TAO's pathogenesis, employing key indicators in our immune study, including cellular immunity, humoral immunization, and immunopathology. Our research unequivocally confirms TAO as an autoimmune disease characterized by multiple hypersensitivity reactions, primarily type III hypersensitivity, accompanied by type II, type IV, and type I reactions. Furthermore, our investigation uncovers a hypercoagulation state in the blood of TAO patients, shedding light on the intricate interplay between vascular immune dysregulation and thrombosis. These insights establish a robust foundation for implication diagnosis and treatment of this complex condition.

Keywords: thromboangiitis obliterans (TAO, Buerger's disease), autoimmune disease, multiple hypersensitivity reactions, hypercoagulation, vascular immune dysregulation, thrombosis, causes of TAO, implications for diagnosis and treatment of TAO

1. Introduction

Buerger's disease (thromboangiitis obliterans, TAO) was first meticulously described by Dr. Leo Buerger in 1908 and 1924. TAO is widely distributed worldwide but exhibits a remarkable variation in incidence worldwide [1]. In North America, it accounts for 0.75%, and in Western Europe, the prevalence ranges from 0.5% to 5.6% of peripheral vascular disease. While in Eastern Europe, the Middle East, the Mediterranean region, and Asia, it accounts for up to 60–80% of peripheral vascular diseases several years ago [1].

TAO is an inflammatory disease affecting the walls of small and medium-sized arteries and veins, accompanied by intraluminal thrombosis, mainly affecting the limbs. The excruciating pain it inflicts has, regrettably, driven some patients toward drug abuse and even limb amputation. In past decades, high-level amputations have soared to an alarming 20% [1]. The severity of the condition underscores its profound implications for public health. Nevertheless, the absence of specific diagnostic markers and the shortage of precise and effective treatment methodologies can be attributed to a limited comprehension of the disease's etiology and pathogenesis. In response, our comprehensive and in-depth investigation into the disease's pathogenesis aims to bridge these gaps in knowledge. We anticipate that our findings will serve as a critical cornerstone in advancing the field.

Given the uneven global distribution of the disease and its infrequent occurrence in certain regions, there remains a pressing need to acquaint medical professionals with its clinical manifestations and diagnosis.

2. Symptoms and signs of TAO

2.1 Abnormal sensation and skin color

The affected extremity may have abnormal sensations like tingling, numbness, or a sensation of burning. The skin color of the affected area can appear pale or purple.

2.2 Coolness

The skin of the affected extremity feels cool to the touch.

2.3 Hair loss or slow hair growth

There may be a loss of hair or reduced hair growth on the affected limb.

2.4 Dry skin and decreased sweating

The skin in the affected area may become dry, and exhibit decreased or no sweating.

2.5 Muscle relaxation, atrophy, and reduced circumference

The muscles in the affected limb may become relaxed, leading to muscle atrophy and a reduced circumference of the limb.

2.6 Migratory superficial phlebitis

More than 50% of cases recur early in TAO or throughout the course of the disease. Painful flushing nodular plaques or cords, mostly located in the superficial veins of the dorsum of the feet and calves, a few cases can extend to the thighs, one or several superficial veins are involved, and the length is several millimeters, several centimeters to several 10 centimeters, the duration of the attack is generally 1–3 weeks, after which the redness, swelling, and pain gradually subside, leaving traces of pigmentation. Some cases have recurrent outbreaks, one after another, more or less, protracted for several years.

2.7 Intermittent claudication

This is a common symptom of TAO. It refers to pain that occurs during physical activity, typically walking. The pain is usually felt in the calf muscles and is often described as a knife-like or colicky sensation. Walking aggravates the pain, and it is relieved by rest. The location of the pain can provide information about the specific arteries that are affected.

2.8 Pain at rest

As TAO progresses, the pain can occur even at rest. It is often more severe when lying down or during sleep. It indicates a severe blockage in the blood vessels, which is a warning of impending ulceration or gangrene in the extremities.

2.9 Ulcers and gangrene

In severe cases of TAO, complete ischemia (lack of blood flow) can lead to the development of ulcers and gangrene in the limb (**Figure 1**). Dry gangrene refers to tissue death without the presence of exudate or pus, while wet gangrene involves tissue infection, edema, and the production of exudate or pus. The pain during this stage is very severe.

2.10 The weakened or disappeared arterial pulses

Mostly in the small and medium arteries. The dorsalis pedis or posterior tibial arteries are the first to be affected by the weakened or disappeared arterial pulses, followed by popliteal and femoral. Iliac arteries and abdominal aorta were very rare. In the upper extremity, the pulsation of the ulnar and radial arteries weakened and disappeared most, followed by the brachial artery, and those involving the axillary artery were very rare.

2.11 Buerger's test positive

The patient lays on his back, raises the lower limbs by 45 degrees for 3 minutes, and performs repeated stretching and flexing of the feet. It can be seen that the skin of the soles of the feet turns pale. Subsequently, the patient experiences increased numbness, coolness, and pain. Guide the patient to sit up and let the lower limbs hung down, resulting in a delayed return of normal skin color to the feet, taking 45–50 seconds (normally within 10 seconds). Additionally, the skin appears excessively flushed.

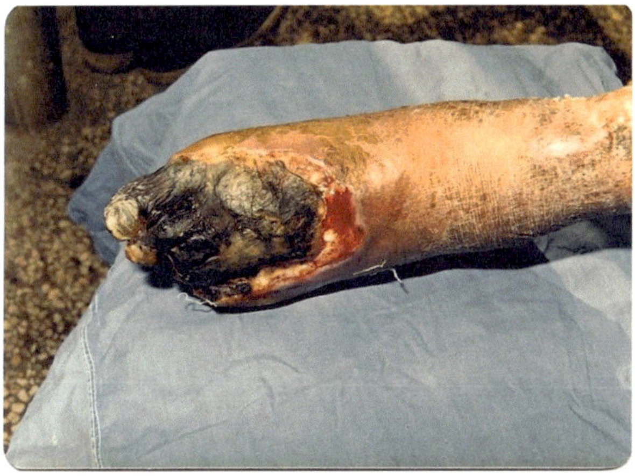

Figure 1.
TAO foot gangrene.

2.12 Clinical manifestations of visceral thromboangiitis obliterans

Visceral TAO is not uncommon [2]. Many scholars have confirmed from autopsy and pathology that the heart (coronary artery), brain (middle cerebral artery and its branches, etc.), and abdominal organs (mesenteric artery, gastroepiploic artery, renal artery, etc.) have the presence of TAO. Clinically, it is seen that some patients with thromboangiitis obliterans with physical symptoms have symptoms of insufficient blood supply to internal organs after several years of onset, such as patients with cerebral artery disease may have migraine, paroxysmal headache, transient hemianopia or amaurosis, transient hemiplegia, sensory impairment, speech impairment, disorientation, memory loss, etc. can also occur.

Patients with coronary artery disease may experience angina pectoris, myocardial infarction, and arrhythmia. Although some cases were confirmed as regressive myocardial infarction by electrocardiogram, the patients were asymptomatic. In some cases, chest tightness and even typical symptoms and signs of myocardial infarction appeared. We have also reported three cases of these kind of patients.

Patients with vascular lesions of the digestive tract may experience paroxysmal abdominal pain, vomiting, diarrhea, and even intestinal necrosis, perforation, and bleeding.

Patients with renal artery disease may experience edema and high blood pressure; urinalysis will show proteinuria, hematuria, and casts.

In short, the symptoms of visceral TAO vary according to the location of the lesion and the degree of obstruction.

3. Clinical diagnostic criteria for TAO of extremities

3.1 The clinical diagnostic criteria for TAO of extremities are as follows

3.1.1 Male predominance

The incidence is mainly in males, with few females. Females should be particularly cautious when diagnosing TAO.

3.1.2 Age of onset

The age of onset is typically between 20 and 40 years old.

3.1.3 Smoking history

The vast majority of patients have a history of smoking.

3.1.4 Superficial phlebitis

Migratory superficial phlebitis in the limbs with a history of recurrent attacks.

3.1.5 Weakening or disappearance of limb artery pulsation

The pulsation of the small arteries in the limbs weakens or disappears, often starting in one lower limb, accompanied by a series of ischemic symptoms such as cold extremities, intermittent claudication, and rest pain.

3.1.6 Exclusion of other vascular diseases

Other vascular diseases caused by different reasons, especially extremity arteriosclerotic occlusion (ASO) and diabetic foot (DF), should be excluded.

3.2 The key points for the diagnosis of visceral thromboangiitis obliterans

3.2.1 Thromboangiitis obliterans

The patient has a history of thromboangiitis obliterans affecting the limbs.

3.2.2 Gradual onset of persistent symptoms

The pathological features usually involve transient ischemic attacks at the onset, which gradually become persistent symptoms.

3.2.3 Rule out other causes of visceral vascular ischemia

Other causes of visceral vascular ischemia should be ruled out.

3.2.4 Arteriography resembling limb TAO arteriography

Visceral arteriography exhibits characteristics similar to limb TAO arteriography.

4. Etiology of Buerger's disease

The etiology of Buerger's disease can be attributed to several factors. Here is a summary of the potential causes identified:

4.1 Age

The onset of Buerger's disease commonly occurs between the ages of 20 and 40, with a majority of cases (84%) falling within this range in our 876 case statistic. It is rare for individuals under the age of 20 to develop the disease. One case of the minimum age is 17 years old in our 876 cases [3].

4.2 Gender

In our analyzed cases, the majority of patients were men, accounting for 99% [3]. However, it is noted that some reports indicate a higher prevalence of the disease in women, potentially linked to an increase in female smokers [1].

4.3 Cold and damp exposure

A significant number of patients had a history of exposure to cold temperatures and humidity before the onset of Buerger's disease. Factors such as sudden exposure to cold after heat during strenuous exercise, as well as exposure to fire after cold, were mentioned. According to our clinical data analysis of this disease, about 80% of the patients had a history of the above condition in 876 cases [3]. It seems that the factors of sudden exposure to cold (heat) and sudden exposure to heat (cold) are very important, which may easily cause vasomotor dysfunction or damage the blood vessels.

4.4 Trauma

While the role of trauma in the development of Buerger's disease requires further clarification, approximately 29% of the patients in the analyzed 876 cases had a history of trauma. Other reports from China suggest a range of 10–35% for trauma-related cases.

4.5 Diet and nutrition

Diet and nutrition: certain dietary factors have been associated with the occurrence of Buerger's disease. Studies have shown a relationship between chronic tobacco poisoning, lack of vitamin B1, and vitamin C deficiency in rats, which can induce vasculitis. Analysis of cases in Indonesia indicated that many patients lacked protein in their diet, particularly essential amino acids. Therefore, nutritional deficiencies may have a connection to the disease's occurrence [4].

4.6 Infection

Some researchers have found dynamic Gram-negative bacilli in the arterial and venous tissue culture fluid of certain Buerger's disease patients. However, the evidence supporting infection, particularly fungal infection, as a significant cause of the disease remains insufficient.

4.7 Smoking

Smoking has been recognized as a primary causative factor in Buerger's disease. Animal experiments using tobacco extract have successfully produced vascular lesions in rats. Skin tests with tobacco extract showed a high positive rate of 78–87% in Buerger's disease patients compared to the general population, which was only 16–46%. According to domestic data, smokers account for 50–95% of the disease, and most of them have a history of heavy smoking. Some patients can improve their condition after quitting smoking, and smoking again can aggravate the symptoms of superficial phlebitis. These show that the onset of the disease is closely related to smoking. Smoking is recognized as the main pathogenic factor of TAO. Not only can smoke be directly sensitized, but nicotine can also be used as a hapten, which binds to histone or DNA in cells, changes the composition of its own tissues, and leads to the production of autoantibodies. Moreover, smoking can also reduce the oxygenation of arterial blood, increase blood viscosity, slow down blood flow, and constrict blood vessels. These phenomena are factors that cannot be ignored in the occurrence and development of vasculitis [5, 6].

Among the 876 cases counted by our hospital, 82% were heavy smokers, but 18% of the cases had never smoked. It shows that smoking is the main factor rather than the only factor.

4.8 Occupation

Workers, peasants, and soldiers accounted for the highest proportion of the number of patients. According to our patients data, they account for about 71–90%.

4.9 Region and race

Initially, the disease was believed to predominantly affect Jews, leading to the term "Jewish disease." Later, it was associated with Eastern European countries, referred to as "Slavic disease" or "Russian disease." However, recent data indicates that Burger's disease can occur in any region and among any nationality. However, the incidence rates vary globally. The prevalence rates among all patients with peripheral arterial diseases have been reported to range from as low as 0.5–5.6% in Western Europe to as high as 45–63% in India. 16–66% in Korea and Japan, and 80% among Ashkenazi Jews [6], Thailand, Indonesia, and Malaysia, all have relatively high incidence rates [1, 7] as well as in China [3]. Recently, the incidence has declined; some authors believe it is related to a decrease in tobacco use, and some authors think it is related to economic development. As for the regional distribution of the disease in China, the disease appears more prevalent in the cold north of China.

4.10 Genetic factors

Some scholars were tested for various HLA antigens. They found that the incidence of HLA-A9 and HLA-B5 was significantly greater among those with Buerger's disease than healthy controls and patients with atherosclerosis [8]. Similarly, in the Merseyside area of the UK, TAO patients exhibited significantly increased levels of HLA-A9 and HLA-B6 antigens. Individuals possessing the HLA-B5 antigen were found to have a relative risk of developing TAO that increased to 78.2 times compared to those without this.

Some scholars observed that HL-A antigen J-1-1 was significantly higher ($P < 0.001$) in Japanese patients with thromboangiitis obliterans (TAO) than it was in a population of normal Japanese. Also, antigens HL-A9 and W10 showed an increased occurrence in TAO patients. However, antigen HL-A12 was not found in TAO patients, but it occurred with a frequency of 20% in the normal population [9]. Some scholars reported patients with TAO had a statistically significantly higher frequency of HLA-DR4 and a significantly lower frequency of the HLA-DRW6 antigen than had both control groups [5].

5. Pathogeneses of Buerger's disease

It is believed immune dysregulation and blood hypercoagulability are very important.

5.1 Autoimmune disease caused by immune regulation disorders

Buerger's disease is an autoimmune disease. And what is the immunological pathogenesis? Over the past 50 years, some scholars have enabled people to have a clearer understanding of the immune pathogenesis of TAO.

In 1962, Pokorny reported that antiarterial antibodies were detected in the blood of TAO patients with superficial migratory phlebitis [10]. Later, some Japanese scholars (1970–1976) obtained results of antiartrial antibodies in almost 50% or more of the patients with TAO. In 1979, Author Ping Zheng postulated that TAO is closely related to the immune mechanism based on the clinical course and pathological manifestation [11]. Culati et al. reported that blood IgG, IgA, and IgM increased, complement CH50 and complement C3 decreased significantly, and the inhibition of leukocyte migration was strengthened in TAO [12]. Later, he reported using indirect fluorescence technology to observe and found anti-IgG, IgA, IgM, and C3 component deposits on the wall of diseased blood vessels—presence of autoantibodies and immune complex in the sera of TAO patients [13, 14]. Bollinger et al. reported that more than 50% of TAO patients had increased antielastin antibodies, decreased complement C4, and 23% of patients had increased blood immune complex CTC [15]; Smolen et al. studied 20 cases of TAO, and detected anticollagen antibodies in seven cases (35%). There was no such antibody in the normal control group [16]. Some scholars have found more antibodies in TAO: antiendothelial cell antibody (AECA), antineutrophil cytoplasmic antibody (ANCA), antiphospholipid antibody (APA), G protein receptor antibody (AAB), etc. [17–21], suggesting that there are many these antibodies attack blood vessel endothelial cells and blood vessel walls.

Also, it has been reported that the role of interleukins [22], cell adhesion molecules [23], and decreased red blood cell immunity [24] on the vascular immune response.

In our study, Since the end of the 1970s, we have conducted comprehensive and systematic research on TAO immunity. We used cellular immunity (T cell rosette test E-RFC, T suppressor cell Ts, peripheral B lymphocytes with SmIg and SmIgG on their surface; leukocyte migration inhibition test, LMIT); humoral immunization (γ-globulin, immunoglobulin IgG, IgA, IgM, IgE, complement CH50, C3, C4, immune complex CIC); and immunopathology (light microscopy, electron microscopy, immunofluorescence IF, immunoenzyme-labeled staining ABC, immune gold and silver staining IGSS), as indicators, systematically observed TAO patients and its immunological changes in acute, subacute, and stable states [25–27].

5.1.1 A summary of our observed immunological changes in TAO patients

5.1.1.1 Cellular immunity

- There is a significant decrease in T cells and Ts ($P < 0.01$), suggesting impaired cellular immune response.
- B cells are increased ($P < 0.01$), indicating an immune response involving antibody production.
- Lymphocytes show degeneration due to aorta antigen sensitization by LMIT.
- LMIT demonstrates enhanced inhibition of leukocyte migration, indicating an immune response.
- Under light microscopy, a large number of lymphocytes, as well as a few monocytes and neutrophils, are observed in all layers of the involved vessels (**Figure 2**).

5.1.1.2 Humoral immunity

- There is a significant increase in the levels of γ-globulin ($P < 0.01$), indicating an immune response.
- Elevated levels of immunoglobulins IgG and IgE are observed ($P < 0.01$).

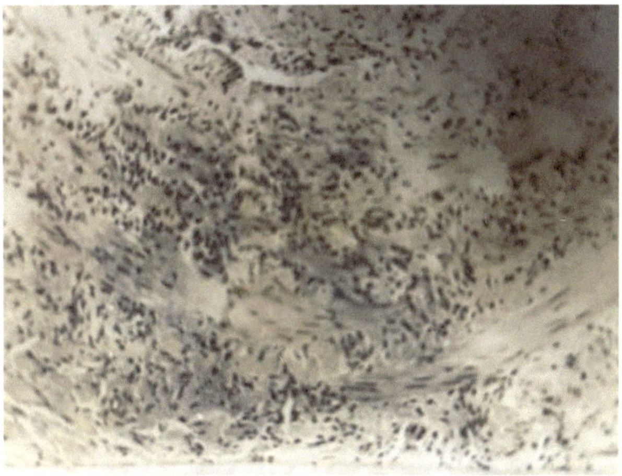

Figure 2.
TAO patient's vein wall thickening and edema, multifocal neutrophil, lymphocytes and a few monocytes, infiltration in the muscle layer, and intravascular thrombus beginning to organize (HE 125×).

- The presence of elevated immune complexes CIC is detected ($P < 0.05$), particularly in the acute stage of TAO ($P < 0.01$), suggesting immune system activation.

- Deposition of immune complexes (CIC) is observed in the blood vessel walls of TAO patients, as confirmed by electron microscopy (**Figure 3**) and three immunolabeling techniques (DIF, ABC, IGSS) (**Figures 4–6**).

- Antivascular autoantibodies are found to directly bind with damaged vascular collagen, as demonstrated by three immunolabeling techniques (**Figures 7–9**).

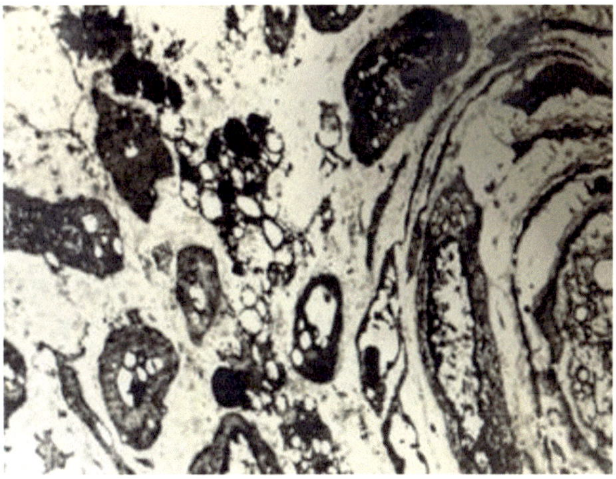

Figure 3.
Deposited with high electronic density lump substance in media corresponding to the area of immunofluorescence deposit in TAO (7490×).

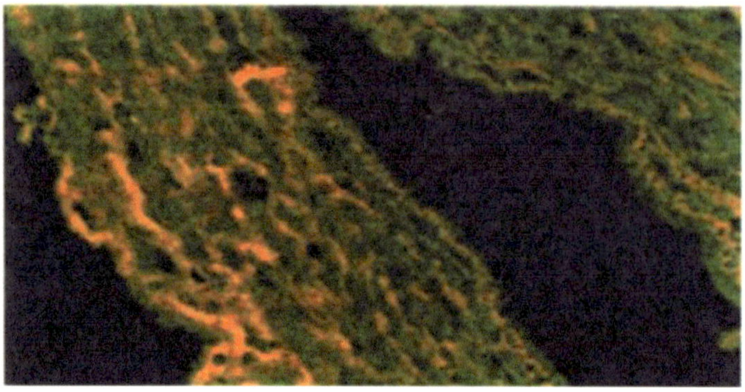

Figure 4.
The deposition of yellow-green striped, plaque-like, and granular immune complex fluorescent substances can be seen in the intima, middle layer, and outer layer of blood vessels of TAO (DIF 400×).

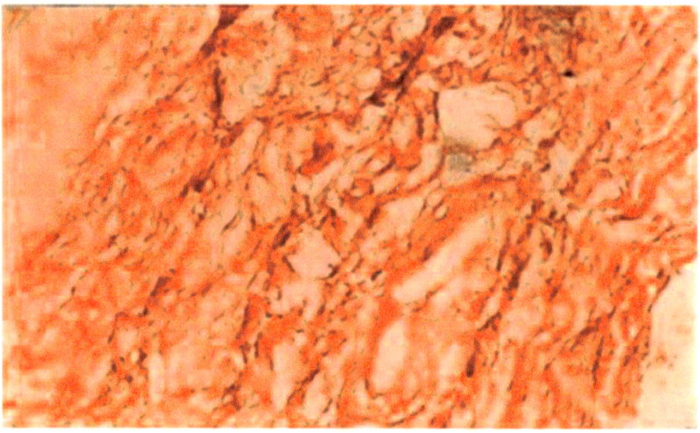

Figure 5.
Streaky and massive brown-yellow immunoenzyme-labeled staining substances deposited on the vessel wall of TAO (ABC 400×).

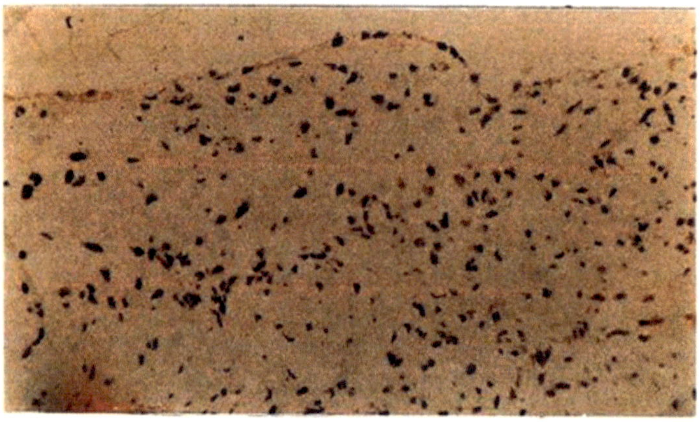

Figure 6.
Black stripes and granular immune gold and silver staining substances were deposited on blood vessels of TAO (IGSS 400×).

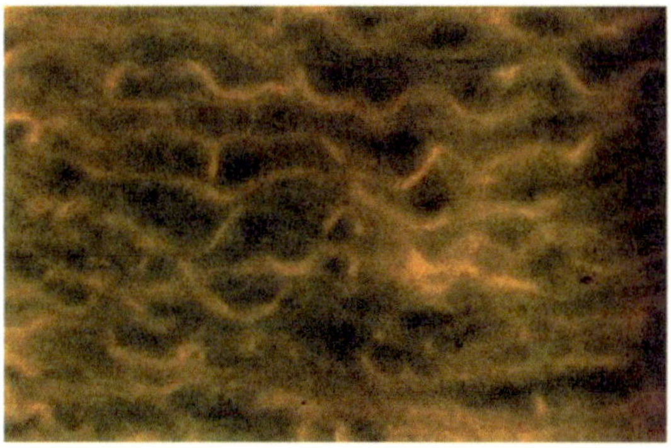

Figure 7.
Antivascular antibodies are present in the sera of TAO patients, showing that the secondary antibody yellow-green FITC-antibody binds to the vessel wall of TAO (DIF 200×).

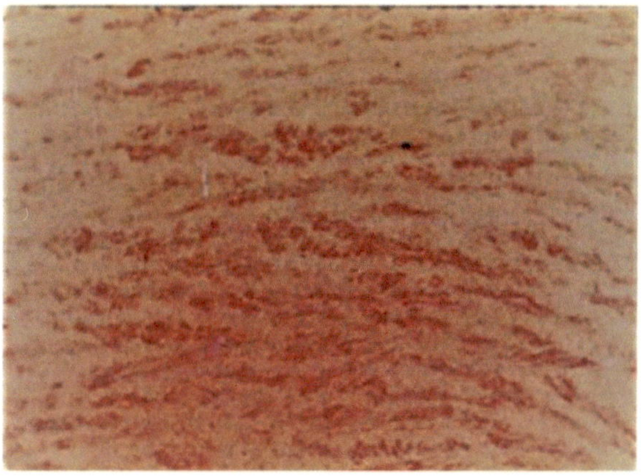

Figure 8.
Antivascular antibodies are present in the sera of TAO patients, showing that the second antibody brown-red antibody binds to the vessel wall of TAO (ABC 200×).

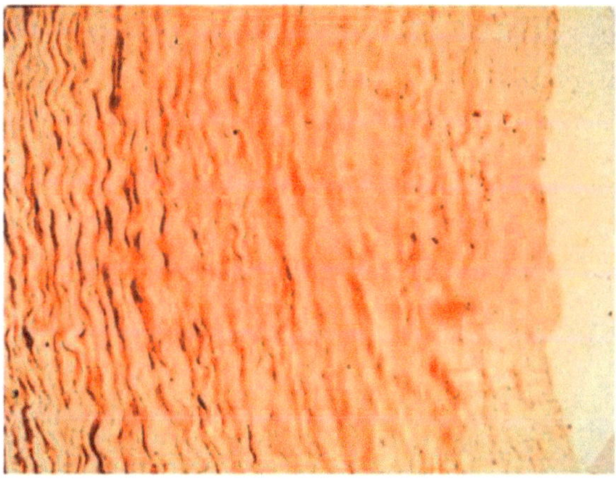

Figure 9.
Antivascular antibodies are present in the sera of TAO patients, showing secondary antibody dark brown gold-antibody bound to the vessel wall of TAO (IGSS 200×).

	Patient group			Normal group			P value
Items	Number of cases	Positive	%	Number of cases	Positive	%	
IF	32	23	72	13	2	18	<0.001
ABC	28	21	75	13	3	23	<0.001
IGSS	28	24	86	11	0	0	<0.001

Table 1.
Detection of antivascular autoantibodies in serum of TAO patients.

- The presence of antivascular autoantibodies in the serum of TAO patients is detected by three immunolabeling techniques, accounting for 72–89% ($P < 0.01$) (**Table 1**).

5.1.2 Conclusions drawn from the provided information

5.1.2.1 Type III hypersensitivity reaction

The presence of antigen-antibody complexes deposited on the vessel wall, confirmed by three immunolabeling techniques and electron microscopy, suggests a type III hypersensitivity reaction in TAO.

5.1.2.2 Type II hypersensitivity

The observation of antivascular autoantibodies directly binding to damaged vascular collagen indicates the existence of type II hypersensitivity in TAO, which was also confirmed by three immunolabeling techniques.

5.1.2.3 Type I hypersensitivity

Elevated levels of IgE and the presence of repeated acute attacks in TAO patients, triggered by factors like tobacco, weather, trauma, and malnutrition, suggest the involvement of type I hypersensitivity. This indicates that the patients may be in a sensitized condition.

5.1.2.4 Type IV delayed hypersensitivity

The results of LMIT show that lymphocytes of TAO patients can be degenerated by aorta antigen sensitization. In light microscopy, lymphocyte infiltration is mainly shown. This, combined with the clinical manifestation of repeated attacks of superficial phlebitis with nodules accompanied by skin inflammation and swelling, suggests the involvement of type IV delayed hypersensitivity. The release of lymphokines by sensitized lymphocytes may contribute to the observed symptoms.

According to clinical studies, patients with TAO have recurrent episodes of superficial phlebitis nodules. The skin on the surface of the nodules is inflammatory and edematous, which may be caused by the release of lymphokines by sensitized lymphocytes. According to light microscopy, lymphocyte infiltration is mainly shown and combined with the results of LMIT. It has also been shown that the lymphocytes of TAO patients can indeed be sensitized by the antigens of the denatured aorta, and the inhibition of leukocyte movement is strengthened.

In summary, TAO appears to involve a combination of type III, type II, type I, and type IV hypersensitivity reactions [25–27].

5.1.3 TAO exhibits characteristics commonly associated with autoimmune diseases

5.1.3.1 Hyperglobulinemia

In TAO, an increase γ-globulin is detected in the blood. γ-globulin is responsible for antibody production, and elevated levels can be observed in various autoimmune diseases.

5.1.3.2 Presence of autoantibodies and sensitized lymphocytes

Autoantibodies are antibodies that mistakenly target and attack the body's own tissues. The presence of autoantibodies and sensitized lymphocytes indicates an immune response against self-antigens, which is a hallmark of autoimmune diseases.

5.1.3.3 Antigen-antibody complexes deposit in damaged tissues

In autoimmune diseases, immune complexes formed by the binding of antigens and antibodies can accumulate in tissues, leading to inflammation and tissue damage.

5.1.3.4 Infiltration of immune cell in target organs

Autoimmune diseases often involve the infiltration of immune cells, such as lymphocytes and monocytes, into the affected organs or tissues.

5.1.3.5 Variety of autoantibodies in TAO patients

The presence of multiple autoantibodies further supports the autoimmune nature of TAO.

5.1.3.6 Genetic predisposition

Like many autoimmune diseases, TAO is also believed to have a genetic component, indicating that certain genetic factors may contribute to its development.

5.1.4 The clinical characteristics of TAO associated with autoimmune diseases

5.1.4.1 Recurrent attacks and chronic protracted process

In our patients with TAO have number of recurrences: one to six times and attack episode duration 1–10 months.

5.1.4.2 Response to immunoadsorption and immunosuppressants during acute attacks

Some researchers have reported that the use of immunoadsorption can help control the progression of TAO disease [28]. Additionally, the author has found that compounds containing immunosuppressive and anticoagulant medications can also effectively manage the development of TAO disease.

5.1.4.3 Presence of TAO in both limbs and internal organs

More and more scholars have reported that TAO not only invades the limbs but also invades visceral blood vessels [29].

5.1.4.4 Association with certain triggering factors

Smoking is recognized as the main pathogenic factor of TAO. Not only can smoke be directly sensitized, but nicotine can also be used as a hapten, which binds to histone or DNA in the cell, changes the composition of its own tissue, and leads to the production of autoantibodies.

5.1.4.5 Changes in sex hormones and autoimmune diseases

Changes in sex hormones can lead to autoimmune diseases [30]. In our cases, 94.5–99% of TAO patients are young and middle-aged men.

5.1.5 In conclusion

Combined, our study identified TAO as an autoimmune disease involving multiple hypersensitivity reactions. Mainly, type III hypersensitivity, in addition to type IV hypersensitivity, also has type II hypersensitivity, and there is the involvement of type I hypersensitivity [25–27].

5.2 TAO blood in hypercoagulable state

In the 1980s, we systematically studied and measured blood hypercoagulation indicators in patients with TAO, including blood coagulation, anticoagulation, platelet function, and blood rheology. We found that out of 14 indicators, 10 exhibited abnormalities [31]:

1. Increased factor VIII-related antigen (VIIIR: Ag) ($P < 0.01$)
2. Decreased antithrombin III (AT-III) ($P < 0.01$)
3. Increased **α**2-macroglobulins (**α** 2-MG) ($P < 0.01$)
4. Increased heparin-precipitated fibrinogen (HPF) ($P < 0.01$)
5. Platelet adhesion rate (PAdT) increased ($P < 0.05$).
6. Platelet aggregation (PAgT) increased ($P < 0.05$, $P < 0.01$)
7. Whole blood and plasma viscosity increased ($P < 0.01$)
8. Red blood cell electric pulse time prolonged ($P < 0.01$)
9. Fibrinogen increased in the disease state ($P < 0.01$)
10. Thromboelastography (TEG) abnormalities

These abnormalities collectively indicate a state of blood hypercoagulability in patients with Buerger's disease, rendering them more susceptible to the formation of thrombi within affected blood vessels. Regarding the relationship between thrombosis and immune-vasculitis in Buerger's disease, it is believed that immune-vasculitis plays a dominant role, and the consequences of various hypersensitivity reactions lead to blood hypercoagulability and thrombosis within the vascular (**Figure 10**).

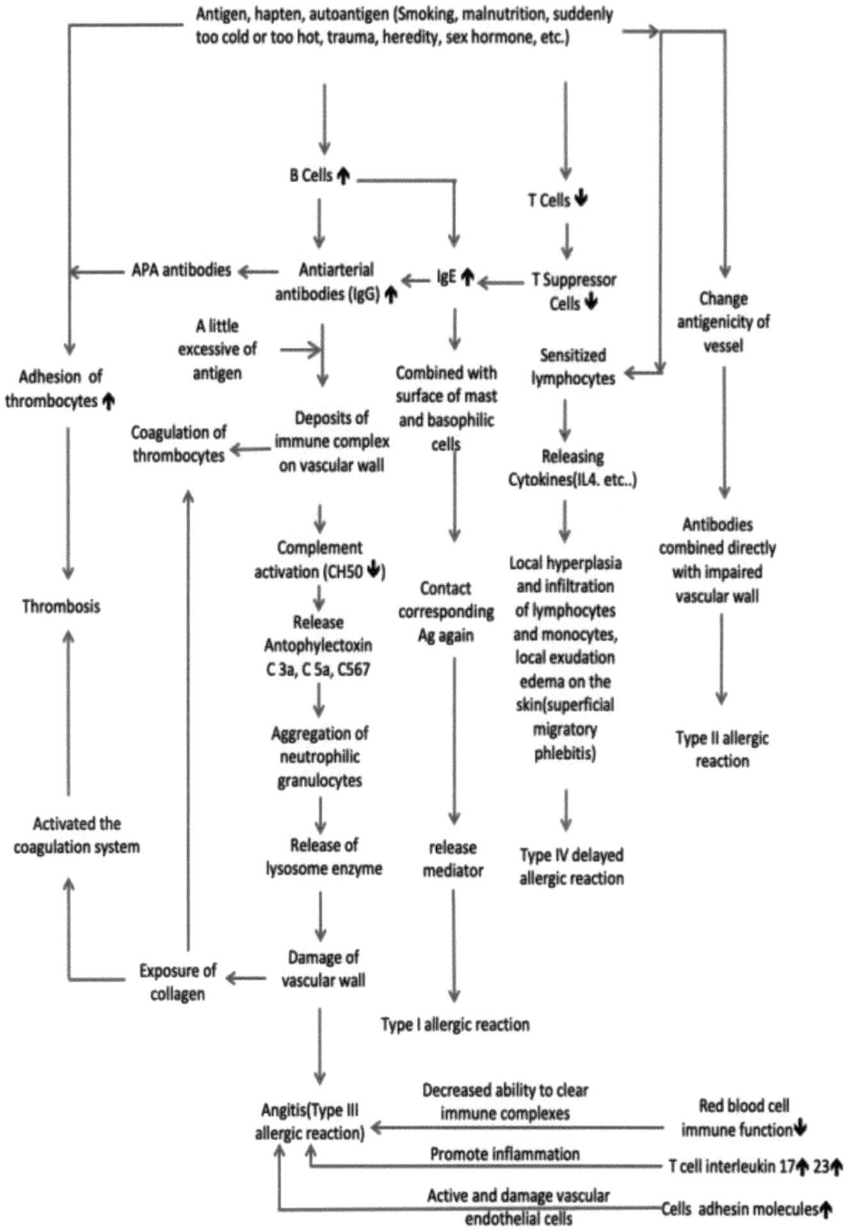

Figure 10.
Conceptual diagram of the pathogenesis of thromboangiitis obliterans (designed by Ping Zheng and Wanchao Wang in 1985, revised in 2020).

6. Implications for diagnosis and treatment of TAO

In the final section of this chapter, we discuss the far-reaching implications of our findings for the diagnosis and treatment of Buerger's disease. Our research provides a solid foundation for the development of diagnostic tools and therapeutic interventions, ultimately improving the outlook for individuals afflicted by this challenging autoimmune disorder.

6.1 Cellular and humoral markers and targeted diagnosis of TAO

The understanding of TAO as a distinct disease separate from other vascular disorders (there is basically no debate among scholars) is relatively recent, dating back about 50 years. Its regional characteristics and varying prevalence in different parts of the world have contributed to slower progress in research. Although the disease is very painful and the amputation rate is high.

In the past four decades, research on the immune pathogenesis of TAO has shifted from scattered detection methods to more comprehensive and in-depth investigations. Scientists have discovered certain cellular and humoral markers associated with the disease.

6.1.1 Cellular markers

Cellular markers refer to specific types of immune cells that are involved in the inflammatory process of TAO. The presence of certain immune cells, such as neutrophils and T lymphocytes, within the affected blood vessels, suggests their role in the disease pathogenesis. Detecting and analyzing these cellular markers can provide insights into the immune response.

6.1.2 Humoral markers

Humoral markers, on the other hand, refer to molecules present in the blood circulation that are associated with the disease. As mentioned earlier, markers such as antivascular antibodies and antigen-antibody complexes have been found to deposit on the walls of blood vessels in TAO. These humoral markers indicate an immune response targeting the vascular endothelium and contribute to the inflammatory process and vessel occlusion seen in the disease.

Furthering efforts to the identification and detection of TAO-specific diagnostic markers from blood circulation are crucial for improving the diagnosis of the disease. By developing reliable and specific tests to detect these markers in the blood circulation, healthcare professionals can potentially diagnose TAO earlier, leading to timely interventions and a reduction in the high amputation rates associated with the disease.

6.2 Treatment of TAO

6.2.1 Avoid triggers of vascular inflammation

Avoid factors that can trigger vascular inflammation, such as nicotine, exposure to sudden cold and sudden heat, and trauma. Smokers should quit smoking immediately and take measures to prevent exposure to temperature extremes and trauma.

DOI: http://dx.doi.org/10.5772/intechopen.1003812

6.2.2 Blocking vascular inflammation and thrombus formation

Appropriate amounts of hormones and anticoagulant drugs can be applied. The author created this kind of compound medicine that has shown promising results without significant side effects. The author has used large doses of anisodamine to

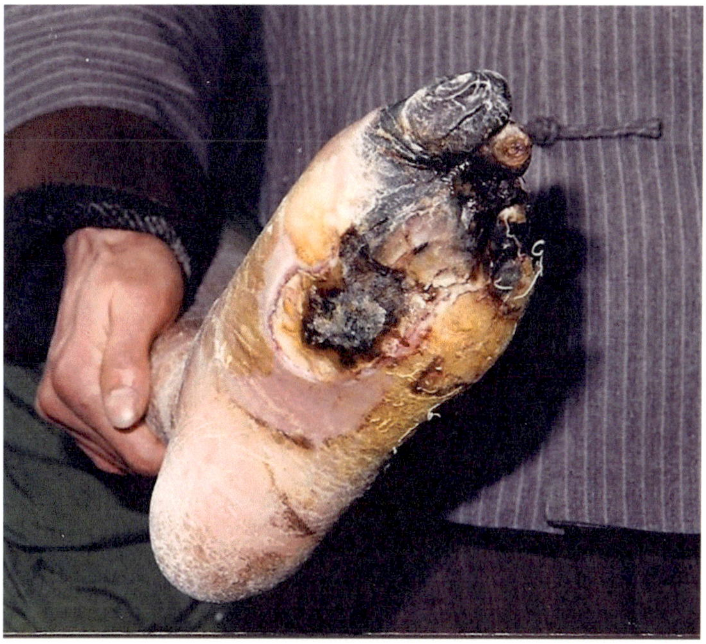

(a)

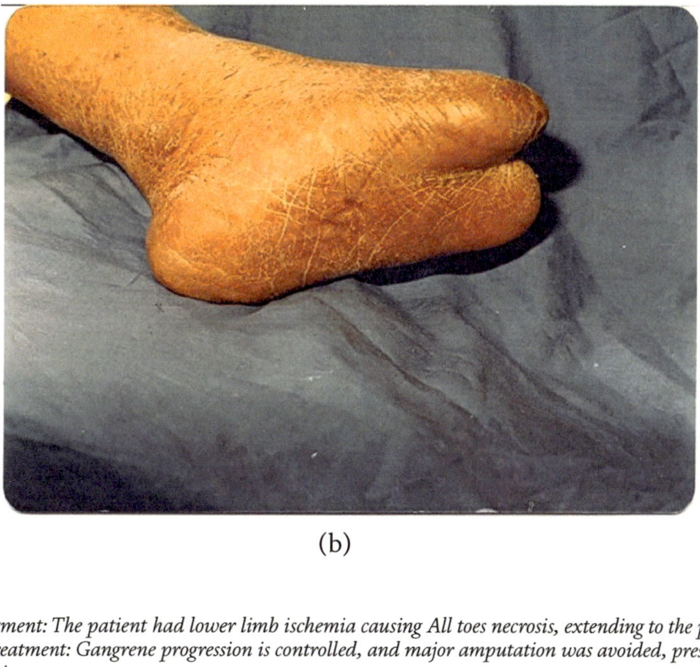

(b)

Figure 11.
(a) Before treatment: The patient had lower limb ischemia causing All toes necrosis, extending to the plantar region. (b) After our treatment: Gangrene progression is controlled, and major amputation was avoided, preserving the heel and plantar region.

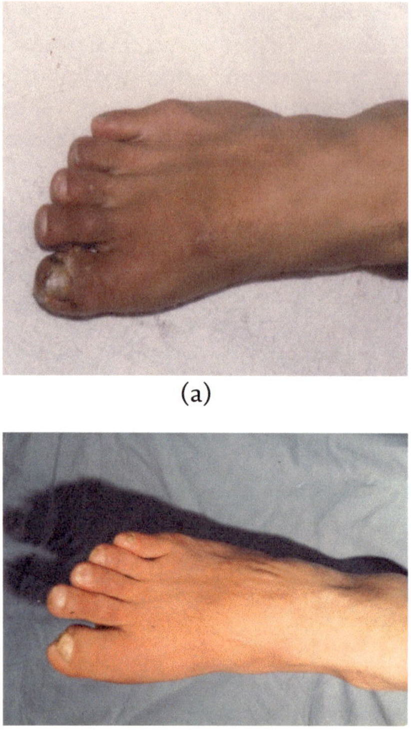

(a)

(b)

Figure 12.
(a) Before treatment: The patient experienced lower limb ischemia resulting in a painful ischemic ulcer on the big toe. (b) After our Treatment: improved limb blood circulation controlled the ulcer's progression, ultimately leading to its complete resolution.

treat TAO in subacute and chronic states, with positive outcomes due to its immune regulation function and ability to reduce blood hypercoagulation [32].

6.2.3 Effective pain relief methods

Effective pain relief is crucial, as severe pain in the affected limb is a major reason for amputation. Anesthesia methods created by the author using a small dose of Traditional Chinese medicine have shown good analgesic effects. This method also promotes blood circulation and regulates immune function. Thereby increasing skin temperature, eliminating limb edema, and improving knee joint flexion deformity [33].

6.2.4 Electroacupuncture

For patients in the subacute or chronic stable stage of TAO, high-frequency electroacupuncture on the affected limbs can improve limb circulation and regulate immune function, leading to increased skin temperature and improved intermittent claudication [34].

Comprehensive treatment combining these above methods can significantly improve therapeutic outcomes, reduce patient pain, and decrease the amputation rate (**Figures 11** and **12**).

Of the 1200 cases we treated, the amputation rate of the thigh and legs above the ankle was 1.2%, and the mortality rate was 0% [35].

7. Conclusion

This chapter's comprehensive exploration of the autoimmune nature of thromboangiitis obliterans (TAO), its intricate involvement of the immune system and secondary blood coagulation pathways, as well as the influences of genetics and the environment, collectively lays a solid foundation for future research endeavors. Moreover, these insights hold significant promise for the advancement of diagnostic techniques and the development of potential therapeutic interventions.

Acknowledgements

We are sincerely grateful to Li Li and YaLi X of the Shanghai Institute of Immunology for their collaboration in some immunological techniques; Professor BaoLi M for her instruction; Professor SaiJuan C of Rui-jin Hospital for TAO blood test cooperation; Professor XueMin T for observing vasseles under eletron microscopy; Professor BinHua S for statistical processing. Dr.JinMing G for assisting in organizing original data.

Conflict of interest

The authors declares that they have no competing interests.

Author details

Ping Zheng[1*] and WanChao Wang[2]

1 Department of Surgery, Ruijin Hospital Affiliated to Shanghai Jiao Tong University, School of Medicine, Shanghai, China

2 Shanghai Institute of Immunology, School of Medicine, Shanghai Jiao Tong University, Shanghai, China

*Address all correspondence to: portiazheng@gmail.com

References

[1] Joseph L, Sr M. Buerger's disease in the 21st century: Diagnosis, clinical features, and therapy. Seminars in Vascular Surgery. 2003;**16**:179-189

[2] Faeze F, Fi B. Visceral bed involvement in thromboangiilis obliterans: A systematic review. Vascular Health and Risk Management. 2019;**15**:317-353

[3] Ping Z. Etiology and pathogenesis of thromboangiitis obliterans (TAO). North Medicine (Chinese). 1983;**5**:13-15

[4] JiaJu W, Zao Wenguang Z, Siqiaoun S, Yang Z. Changes in the incidence of thromboangiitis obliterans. Chinese Journal of Vascular Surgery. 2009;**1**:9-12

[5] Papa M, Bass A, Adar R, Halperin Z, Schneiderman J, Becker CG, et al. Autoimmune mechanisms in thromboangiitis obliterans (Buerger's disease): The role of tobacco antigen and the major histocompatibility complex. Surgery. 1992;**111**(5):527-531

[6] Abhishek V, Rahul T, Vinod KP. Thromboangiitis obliterans (Buerger's disease)—Current practices. International Journal of Inflammation. 2013;**2013**:156905. DOI: 10.1155/2013/156905. Epub 2013 Sep 11

[7] Peter F, Lein-Weigel K, Richer JG. Thromboangiitis obliterans (Buerger's disease). VASA. 2014;**43**:337-350

[8] McLoughlin GA, Helsby CR, Evans CC, Chapman D. Association of HLA—A9 and HLA—B5 with Buerger's disease. British Medical Journal. 1976;**2**:1165-1166

[9] Ohtawa TT, Kawano N, Mishima Y, Tohyama H, Ishikawa K. HLA antigens in thromboangiitis obliterans. Journal of the American Medical Association. 1974;**230**(8):1128

[10] Pokorny J, Jezkova Z. Significance of immunological studies in peripheral obliterating vascular diseases. Circulation Research. 1962;**11**(6):961

[11] Ping Z. Treatment and prevention on TAO with Chinese traditional medicine combine with Western medicine. Compiled per TAO Experience Exchange Symposium (Chinese). Ji Nan China. 1976:125-133

[12] Gulati SM, Madhar K, Thusoo TK, Nair SK, Saha K. Immunological studies in thromangiitis obliterans (Buerger's disease). The Journal of Surgical Research. 1979;**27**:287

[13] Gulati SM, Madhar TK, Nair SK, Saha K. Autoantibidies in thromboangiitis obliterans (Buerger's disease). Angiology. 1982;**33**(10):642-651

[14] Gulati SM, Saha K, Kant L, Thsoo TK, Prakash A. Significance of circullatory immune complexes in thromboangiitis obliterans (Buerger's disease). Angiology. 1984;**35**(5):276-281

[15] Bollinger A, Piquerez MJ, Largiader J, Schneider E. Buerger's disease present diagnostic and therapeutic method. Annales de Médecine Interne. 1983;**134**(5):436-440

[16] Adar R, Papa MZ, Halpern Z. Cellular sensitivity to collagen in thromboangiitis obliterans. New England Medicine. 1983;**308**(19):1113-1123

[17] Eichhorn J, Sima D, Lindschau C, Turowski A, Schmidt H, Schneider W, et al. Antiendothelial cell antibodiin

thromboangiitis obliterans. The American Journal of the Medical Sciences. 1998;**315**:17-23

[18] Halacheva KS, Manolova IM, Petkov DP, Andreev AP. Study of anti-neutrophil cytoplasmic antibodies in patients with thromboangiitis obliterans (Buerger's disease). Scandinavian Journal of Immunology. 1998;**48**:544-550

[19] Maslowski L, McBane R, Alexewicz P, Wysokinski WE. Antiphospholipid antibodies in thromboangiitis obliterans. Vascular Medicine. 2002;7:259-264

[20] de Godoy JM, Braile DM. Buerger's disease and anticardiolipin antibodies. Journal of Cardiovascular Medicine. 2009;**10**:792-794

[21] Klein-Weigel PF, Bimmler M, Hempel P, Schöpp S, Dreusicke S, Valerius J, et al. G-protein coupled receptor auto-antibodies in thromboangiitis obliterans (Buerger's disease) and their removal by immunoadsorption. VASA. 2014;**43**:347-352

[22] Dellalibera-joviliano R, Joviliano EE, Silva JS, Evora PR. Activation of cytokines corroborate with development of inflamation and autoimmunity in thromboangiitis oblierans patients. Clinical & Experimental Immunology. 2012;**170**:28-35

[23] Zheng W, Wenjing J, Hengzhen W, Li H, Bo T, Bing L, et al. The IL-6/Stat3 pathway regulates adhesion molecules and cytoskeleto endothelial cell in throboangiitis obliterans. Cellular Signalling. 2016;**44**:118-126. DOI: 10.1016/j.cellsig.2018.01.015

[24] Xiangmao F, Zaiping J, Feng G. Erythrocyte immune function and regulatory factors in patients with thromboangiitis obliterans (Chinese). Shanghai Medicine. 1987;**20**:403-404

[25] Ping Z, PeiBing F, Wang W, WunYu X, Ton XM, Ming Y, et al. Observation on the immune function status of thromboangiitis obliterans (Chinese). Journal of Shanghai Immune. 1985;**5**(3):146-150

[26] Ping Z, PeiBin F, Wang W, WenYu X, XueMing T, Ming Y, et al. Immunological studies on thromboangiitis obliterans. Chinese Medical Journal. 1989;**102**(2):129-136

[27] Ping Z, Wang W. Buerger's disease: Autoimmune disease involving multiple hypersensitivity types. Journal of Clinic Research. 2022;**6**:S1

[28] Bauman G, Verena S, Peter KW, Karl S. Successful treatment of throboangiitis obliterans (Buerger's disease) with immunoadsorption: Results of a pilot study. Clinical Research in Cardiology. 2011;**100**:683-690

[29] Ping Z, LiNian Z. Thromboangiitis obliterans with myocardial infarction in 3 case. Cardiovascular Diseases. 1978;**6**:19-21

[30] Sun K, Feng Q, Dou K. The relationship between the immunomodulatory effects of sex hormones and the occurrence of diseases (Chinese). Chinese Journal of Preventive Medicine. 2002;**36**(6):421-423

[31] Ping Z, SaiJuan C, HaiZheng C. Studies on hypercoagulation state in Buerger's disease. Chinese Medical Journal. 1989;**102**(1):67-71

[32] Ping Z. High-dose anisodamine in the treatment of 62 cases of thromboangiitis obliterans (Chinese). Chinese Emergency Medicine. 1990;**10**(1):3-6

[33] Ping Z. Traditional Chinese medicine anesthesia in severe thromboangiitis obliterance. Chinese Medical Journal. 1988;**101**(3):221-224

[34] Ping Z. Thromboangiitis obliterans (Chinese). In: Zhenyi W, editor. Thrombosis and Hemostasis. Shanghai of China: Shanghai Science and Technology Press; 1988. pp. 246-254. ISBN:7-5323-0346-2

[35] Ping Z. Comprehensive treatment of thromboangiitis obliterans with integrated Traditional Chinese and Western medicine (Chinese). In: The Ninth National Surgery Academic Conference. Wu Han, China 1978 Proceedings of Abstract. p. 19

Chapter 6

Perspective Chapter: Role of Anti-TPO Association with the Autoimmune Thyroid Diseases

Nurakant Neupane

Abstract

An organization of cells and molecules with specific functions for protection against infection is known as the immune system. When immune system reacts against its own cells known as an autoimmune disease. Autoimmune thyroid diseases are grouped under endocrinal diseases in which the immune system attacks the body's own thyroid gland. In autoimmune thyroid disease (AITD), an immunological alteration occurs in the follicular cells of the thyroid gland. In this case, certain enzymes, surface proteins, and receptors such as thyroperoxidase, thyroglobulin, and thyroid-stimulating hormone (TSH) receptors start acting as antigens; against these antigens, relevant antibodies are produced by the body, and cell-mediated cytotoxicity gets induced. These autoimmune endocrinal diseases are characterized by the presence of high titers of antibodies like thyroperoxidase antibodies (TPO-Abs) and thyroglobulin antibodies, produced by our own body system. In conclusion, anti-TPO can play a crucial role in the diagnosis of autoimmune thyroiditis. Anti-TPO is the prognosis marker for the child and adult who have normal thyroid function tests in euthyroidism, subclinical thyroidism. Thus, anti-TPO along with thyroid function tests play a substantial role in the clinical management of autoimmune thyroiditis.

Keywords: autoimmune thyroid disease, anti-TPO, endocrine, immune system, thyroid gland

1. Introduction

Immune system is made up of complex organ systems, cells, and proteins to fight against pathogens (microbes). This immune system helps to keep the body healthy by protecting fight against pathogens. Defects in the immune system or malfunctioning in the immune response can provoke illness or disease. When the immune systems reacts against self-cells is known as autoimmune disease. These autoimmune diseases are either organ-specific or systemic disease. Autoimmune thyroiditis is organ-specific autoimmune disease.

Autoimmune thyroid diseases are grouped under endocrinal diseases in which the immune system attacks the body's own thyroid gland. These autoimmune endocrinal diseases are characterized by the presence of high titers of antibodies, such as TPO-Abs (thyroperoxidase antibodies) and thyroglobulin antibodies, produced by our own body system.

Due to the organ-specific autoimmune disorders, autoimmune thyroid disease is much more common in women than men [1]. Men are affected by 1%, whereas women are by 2–4%, which rate surges with age worldwide [2].

Hereditary factors, that is, gene alteration are one of the main causes in manifestation of AITD, and other factors such as advancing age, smoking, iodine overconsumption, adverse effects of medication, and hormonal changes (in females) known as environmental and endogenous are also responsible for the initiation of AIDT [3, 4].

In AITD, immunological alteration occurs in the follicular cells of the thyroid gland. In this case, certain enzymes, surface proteins, and receptors such as thyroperoxidase, thyroglobulin, and TSH receptors start acting as antigen; against these antigens, relevant antibodies are produced by the body, and cell-mediated cytotoxicity gets induced. This leads to autoimmune thyroid disease. These antibodies damage the thyrocytes and cause inflammation of the thyroid gland [4, 5].

The common antibodies measured in serum samples are thyroglobulin and thyroperoxidase antibodies [5]. TPO antibody has frequently been found in the general population as compared to other antibodies. Along with TSH, free T_3 and free $T_{4,}$ anti-TPO antibodies are more specific in the diagnosis of AITD. The levels of free T_3, free $T_{4,}$ and TSH help in distinguishing the two conditions: hypothyroidism and hyperthyroidism. Hypothyroidism is a condition in which the level of thyroid hormones (free T_3, free T_4 decreases), and in hyperthyroidism, the level of thyroid hormones increases from its normal range. The titer of anti-TPO antibodies above its normal value indicates an autoimmune response to the thyroid gland. So, anti-TPO antibody testing is helpful in differentiating between autoimmune thyroid disease and other thyroid disorders.

Thyroid diseases are classified as euthyroidism, subclinical thyroidism, and clinical or overt thyroidism on the basis of thyroid hormone levels. Anti-TPO antibody, TSH, free T_3, and free T_4 remain normal in euthyroidism. In subclinical thyroidism, anti-TPO antibodies and TSH are increased and patients remain asymptomatic with mild impairment in the thyroid gland. It is more common than overt thyroidism, and it can prevent the progression of overt thyroidism and have effects on early diagnosis and treatment of subclinical thyroidism [6]. Anti-TPO Abs and TSH are remarkably increased in overt thyroidism, whereas other thyroid hormones' levels depend upon hyperthyroidism or hypothyroidism. Clinical thyroiditis is a symptomatic disease and depression, unexplained weight loss, etc. are the main complications. Hashimoto and graves' thyroid diseases are common examples. In this chapter, we will discuss a brief introduction of immune system and its type and a detail discussion of autoimmune thyroiditis, the role of anti-TPO in autoimmune thyroiditis, and the clinical application of anti-TPO in diagnosis and management of autoimmune disease.

2. Method

The following databases were thoroughly search: Web of Science, Scopus, PubMed/MEDLINE, Google scholar, Sematic Scholar, Embase. The terms autoimmune thyroiditis, Hashimoto thyroiditis, Graves' disease, and anti-TPO were used in a search for articles that had no specific publication date.

3. Immune system

An organization of cells and molecules with a specific function for protection against infection is known as immune system. Basically, there are two types of immune responses, that is, innate immunity and adaptive immunity to intruding microbes (organisms such as bacteria, fungi, and parasites), viruses, cancer cells, and toxins. Innate (natural) immune system is the first line of defense for invading pathogens also known as the non-specific immune system, whereas the adaptive (acquired) immune system is the second line of defense response to repeated exposure to microbial antigens during the innate immune. Phagocytic cells (neutrophils, monocytes, and macrophages) use innate responses that release (basophils, mast cells, and eosinophils), and natural killer cells as inflammatory mediators. Complement, acute-phage proteins, and cytokines-interferons- are the molecular component of innate immunity. Proliferations of antigen-specific B and T cells are mainly involved in the acquired immune system and this occurs when an antigen binds to the surface receptors of these cells. In the response of the antigen, antigen-presenting cells display to lymphocytes and collaborate with them. The production of antibodies by B cells is helped by T cells, which may also kill virally infected cells and destroy intracellular infections by activating macrophages. Pathogens are typically eliminated together by the responses of innate and acquired. **Figure 1** shows the principal characteristics of innate and adaptive immunity and innate and adaptive immune responses [7, 8].

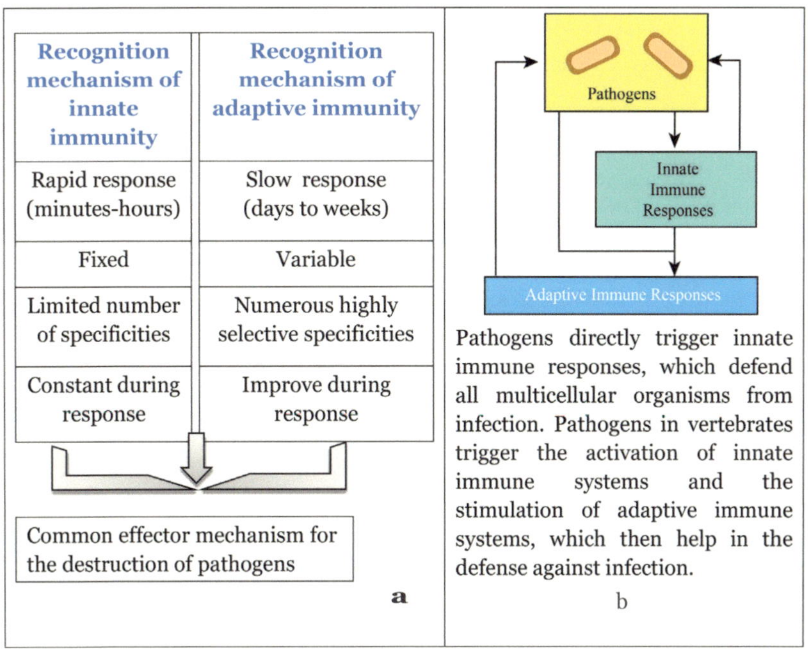

Figure 1.
(a) The principal characteristics of innate and adaptive immunity. (b). Innate and adaptive immune responses [7, 8].

3.1 Innate immunity

Within minutes or hours of coming into contact with an antigen, the host activates innate immunity, a non-specific (antigen-independent) defensive mechanism. Since the innate immune system lacks immunologic memory, it is unable to identify or "memorize" the same pathogen should the body come into contact with it again in the future. Four different forms of protective barriers are included in innate immunity: anatomic (skin and mucous membrane), physiological (temperature, low pH, and chemical mediators), endocytic and phagocytes, and inflammatory. The barrier of non-specific host-defense mechanisms is summarized in **Table 1**. Innate immunity to infections is dependent on pattern recognition receptors (PRRs), which enable a specific subset of immune cells to quickly identify and react to a variety of pathogens that have similar molecular patterns (PAMPs). These include bacterial cell walls such as lipopolysaccharides (LPS) and double-stranded ribonucleic acid (RNA) generated during viral infection.

3.2 Adaptive immunity

The adaptive immune responses are very specific to the individual pathogen that triggered them, in contrast to innate immune responses. Additionally, they can provide enduring defense. The adaptive immune system, for instance, provides lifelong immunity against measles for those who have recovered from the disease,

Barrier	Mechanism
Anatomic	
Skin	• Mechanical barrier retards entry of microbes • Acidic environment (pH 3–5) retards growth of microbes
Mucous membrane	• Normal flora compete with microbes for attachment sites • Mucous entraps foreign microbes • Cilia propel microbes out of body
Physiologic	
Temperature	Body temperature/fever response inhibits growth of some pathogens
Low pH	Acidic pH of stomach kills most undigested microbes
Chemical mediators	• Lysozyme cleaves bacterial cell wall • Interferon induces antiviral defenses in uninfected cells • Complement lyses microbes or facilitates phagocytosis
Phagocytic/endocytic barriers • Various cells internalize (endocytosis) and break down foreign macromolecules • Specialized cells (blood monocytes, neutrophils, tissue macroph	
Inflammatory barriers • Tissue damage and infection induce leakage of vascular fluid containing serum protein with antibacterial activity, leading to influx of phagocytic cells into the affected area	

Table 1.
Summary of non-specific host-defense mechanism for barriers of innate immunity.

but not to other common viruses like those that cause mumps or chickenpox. Recognition of particular "non-self" antigens and their distinction from "self" antigens; development of pathogen-specific immunologic effector pathways that destroy particular pathogens or pathogen-infected cells; and the formation of an immunologic memory that can quickly eradicate a specific pathogen should consequent infections occur are the three main functions of an adaptive immune response [9]. Adaptive immune responses are the basis for effective immunization against infectious diseases. The cells of the adaptive immune system include antigen-specific T cells, which are activated to proliferate through the action of APCs, and B cells which differentiate into plasma cells to produce antibodies. Effective immunization against infectious illnesses is based on adaptive immune responses. The cells of the adaptive immune system are antigen-specific T cells and B cells. T cells are activated to proliferate through the action of APCs, and B cells differentiate into plasma cells to produce antibodies. Activation and function of B cells and T cells are summarized in **Figure 2** [10]. Apart from this, B cells play a major role in the humoral or antibody-mediated immune response and T cells play the cell-mediated immune response [9, 11].

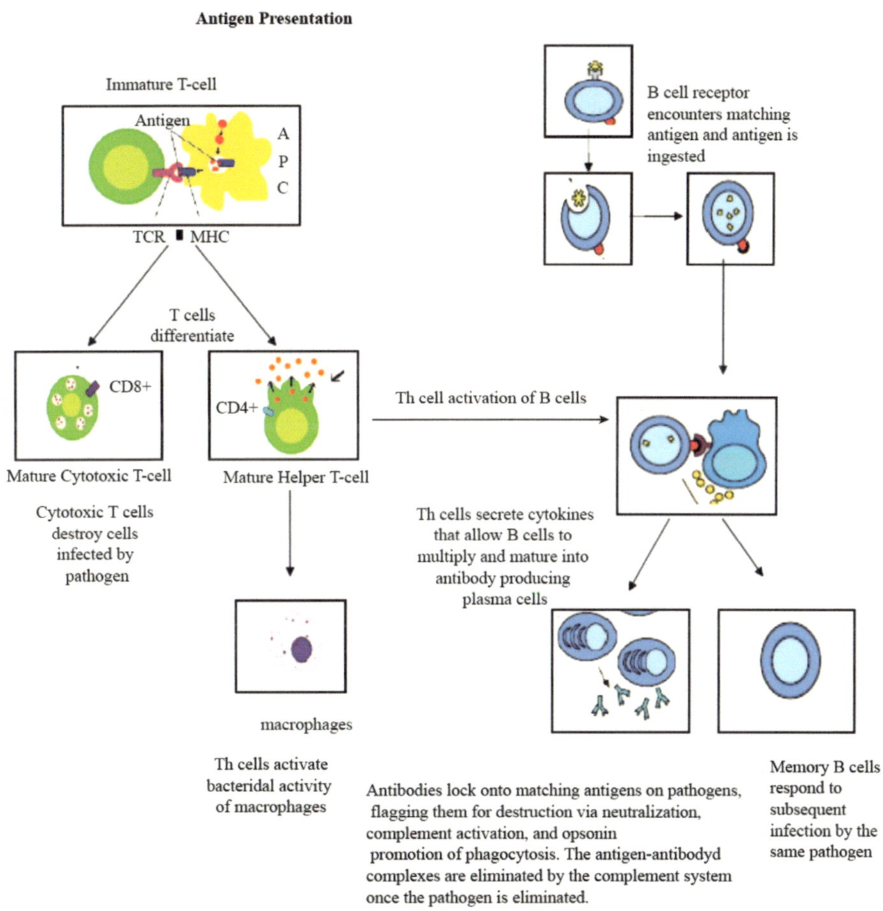

Figure 2.
Adaptive immunity: T-cell and B-cell activation and function [10].

3.3 Antibody-mediated and cell-mediated immunity

3.3.1 Antibody-mediated immunity

The immunity mediated by B-cell-antibody production in the extracellular body fluids in the responses of pathogen is known as antibody-mediated or humoral immunity. When the B cell's antigen-binding receptor recognizes and attaches to antigen in its native form, the antibody production pathway begins. Local Th cells release cytokines that support B cell proliferation and direct the type of antibody generated. Certain cytokines, such as IL-6, aid in the maturation of B-cells into antibody-secreting plasma cells. Secreted antibodies attach to antigens on pathogen surfaces, signaling them for destruction via complement activation, opsonin-mediated phagocytosis, and pathogen elimination by immune effector cells. The complement cascade clears antigen-antibody complexes after the pathogen is eliminated. Therefore, antibody-mediated immunity plays an important role against pathogens that grow on extracellular spaces. The basic model of antibody-mediated immunity against pathogens (virus) is shown in **Figure 3** [12].

B cells produce five major types of antibodies: IgA, IgD, IgE, IgG, and IgM. IgG antibodies can be further split into structurally diverse subclasses with a range of complement fixing, opsonin, and other functional properties. The major classes of antibodies recognize and neutralize specific pathogens that have substantially different biological functions [10].

During the acute stage of infection, antibodies are crucial in controlling viral growth. However, once a virus has been infected, they are typically unable to remove it.

3.3.2 Cell-mediated immunity

When an infection is established, cell-mediated immune mechanisms are significant in host defense against most intracellular pathogens. Cell-mediated immunity is other

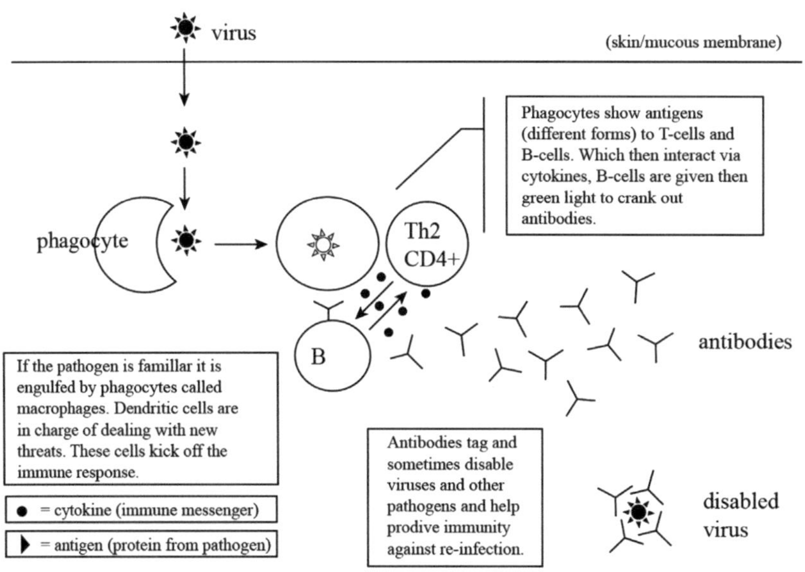

Figure 3.
Basic model of antibody-mediated (Th_2) immunity against pathogen [12].

kind of adaptive immunity that generates mature T cells, macrophages, and cytokines against pathogens are proliferated. In addition, two types of lymphocytes are engaged in cell-mediated immunity: helper T cells and cytotoxic T cells. The cell-mediated immunity proceeds in three phases including T-cell activation by presenting antigens with MHC complexes, T-cell binding and activation, and differentiation of activated T cells into effector cells and memory T cells, which is illustrated in **Figure 4** [12].

Furthermore, T cells are generated in the bone marrow and mature in the thymus. T cells are found in the blood and lymphoid tissue after entering the bloodstream. Antigen-presenting cells (APCs) present antigens to T lymphocytes together with major histocompatibility complexes (MHC). T cells proliferate and develop into armed effector cells when they come into contact with an antigen. Cytotoxic T cells kill infected cells by triggering apoptosis. T helper cells encourage the production of antibodies by plasma B cells.

In addition, IgG and IgM antibodies are the two main types of antibodies produced by T helper cells in response to plasma B cells. Memory T cells are developed T cells, but their action is dependent on antigen activation. Cellular immunity is most effective against virus-infected cells and cancer cells, but it can also help to guard against fungus, protozoa, malignancies, and intracellular bacteria. This type of immunity also plays a significant role in transplant rejection.

3.4 Active and passive immunity

3.4.1 Active immunity

When the immune system produces antibodies to a disease after being exposed to the disease organism is known as active immunity. Either natural immunity or vaccine-induced immunity can be used to build up active immunity.

- Exposure to the disease agent and subsequent infection with the disease itself are the two ways that natural immunity is acquired.

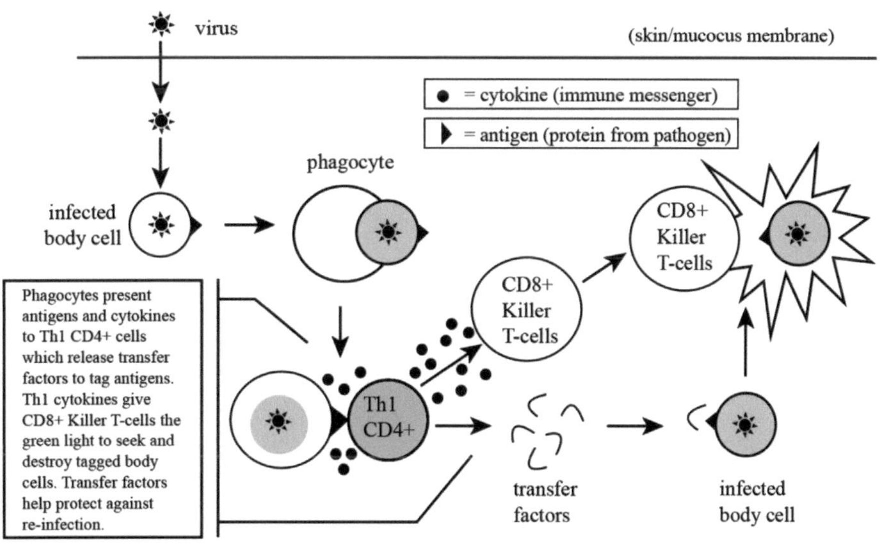

Figure 4.
Basic model of cellular-mediated (Th1) immunity with pathogen (virus) [12].

- Vaccine-induced immunity is acquired through the administration of a vaccine that can consist of attenuated (weakened) pathogens, inactivated organisms or specific proteins, or carbohydrates known to induce immunity.

In any case, if an immune individual later comes into contact with that disease, their immune system will instantly recognize it and produce the antibodies required to fight it. Active immunity lasts for a very long time—sometimes a lifetime.

3.5 Passive immunity

When an antibody against a disease is given to a person rather than the individual making them naturally through their immune system is called passive immunity.

- Through the placenta, a newborn baby gains passive immunity from its mother.

- By receiving immune globulin or other blood products containing antibodies, such as those used to treat specific diseases, people can potentially develop passive immunity.

The main benefit of passive immunity is that it provides protection immediately, in contrast to active immunity, which takes time (often several weeks) to develop. However, passive immunity only lasts a few weeks or months. Long-lasting can only be active immunity.

3.6 Immunopathology

Defects or malfunctions in either the innate or adaptive immune response can provoke illness or disease. Such disorders are generally caused by an overactive immune response (known as hypersensitivity reactions), ineffective immune responses (known as immunodeficiency), or an inappropriate reaction to self (known as autoimmunity).

3.6.1 Hypersensitivity reactions

An undesirable responses produced by the normal immune system are referred to as hypersensitivity reactions. There are four types of hypersensitivity reactions [13, 14].

- Type I: immediate hypersensitivity

- Type II: cytotoxic or antibody-dependent hypersensitivity

- Type III: immune complex disease

- Type IV: delayed-type hypersensitivity

3.6.2 Immunodeficiency

When the ability to fight against infectious disease is compromised or totally absent is known as immunodeficiency. Immunodeficiency can be caused by a mainly genetic defect (primary immunodeficiency), which can affect innate or acquired immune function by inhibiting specific immune cells or pathways, or they can develop as a result of a secondary cause (secondary immunodeficiency), such as bacterial or viral infections, malnutrition, autoimmunity, or medication that causes immunosuppression. Leukemia and multiple myeloma are immunodeficiency disorders that directly or indirectly impair the immune system. Immunodeficiency is also the hallmark of acquired immunodeficiency syndrome (AIDS), caused by the human immunodeficiency virus (IV). HIV directly infects Th cells and also weakens other immune system responses [15, 16].

3.6.3 Autoimmunity

Autoimmune disease is characterized by the activity of auto-reactive lymphocytes, which cause loss of normal immune homeostasis that react against host tissues, or effector T cells, which are specific for endogenous self-peptides [17]. The presence of self-reactive T cells, auto-antibodies, and inflammation are the main characteristics of autoimmunity. Autoimmune diseases can be classified as either systemic or organ-specific. In systemic disease, the immune system attacks self-antigen in several organs. For instance, in systemic lupus, erythematous inflammation occurs in several organs, such as the skin, joints, and kidneys, among other organs. In an organ-specific disease, the immune response is directed toward antigens in a single organ. For example, autoantibodies attack the adrenal cortex in Addison's disease. Some common examples of autoimmune diseases are Celiac disease, type 1 diabetes mellitus, Addison's disease, and autoimmune thyroiditis [18]. In autoimmune thyroiditis immune system attacks on the thyroid gland cause disorders in thyroid hormones consequences effects on the metabolic system, body temperature, and proteins synthesis, etc.

4. Thyroid gland

The thyroid gland is an endocrine gland located in the neck region, in front of the larynx and trachea. Leonardo Da Vinci was the first scientist to draw the thyroid gland as an anatomical organ [19]. Andreas Vesalius, an anatomist, published the first anatomic description and image of the gland in 1543. Thyroid Wharton, in 1656, used the term "thyroid" for the first time [20]. Thyroid is a Greek word to indicate the shape of a shield. In 1656, the thyroid gland was mentioned in Western medicine for the first time; before this, it was considered to have lubrication of trachea as its main function [21]. The thyroid gland contains numerous follicles, composed of epithelial follicle cells and colloids [22]. The main function of the thyroid gland is to make major hormones like T_3 and T_4 required for the maintenance and regulation of metabolic processes throughout the body. An endocrinal disease of thyroid gland leads to under or overproduction of these hormones due to adverse activity of the gland. AIDT is one of the major endocrinal diseases in which antibodies are produced against the own thyroid cells, i.e., thyrocytes, and inflammation of the thyroid gland occurs [23].

As shown in **Figure 5**, the thyroid gland produces mainly two hormones, T_3 (tri-iodotyrosine) and T_4 (tetra-iodotyrosine) [24]. The synthesis of these two hormones takes place in the follicular cells of the thyroid gland. The process is regulated by the hypothalamus, the master gland, and by feedback inhibition mechanism [25]. The mechanisms of biosynthesis of thyroid hormones are illustrated below:

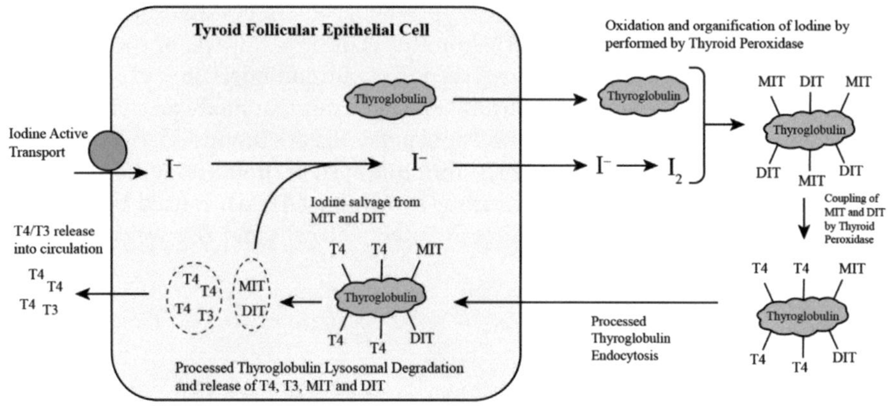

[Source:- https://rushem.org/2018/12/19/thyroid-emergencies-in-a-rush/]

Figure 5.
Synthesis of thyroid hormones [24].

- Uptake of iodide by follicular cells.
- Iodine organification by thyroperoxidase.
- Combining of iodine and thyroglobulin.
- MIT (Mono-Iodotyrosine) /DIT (Di-Iodotyrosine) store in follicular space.
- Reabsorbing of MIT/DIT.
- T_3, T_4 formation from MIT/DIT.
- T_3, T_4 release into serum.
- With the release of iodine T_3, T_4 break down.

Biochemical structure of T_3 and T_4 is shown below in **Figure 6** [26].

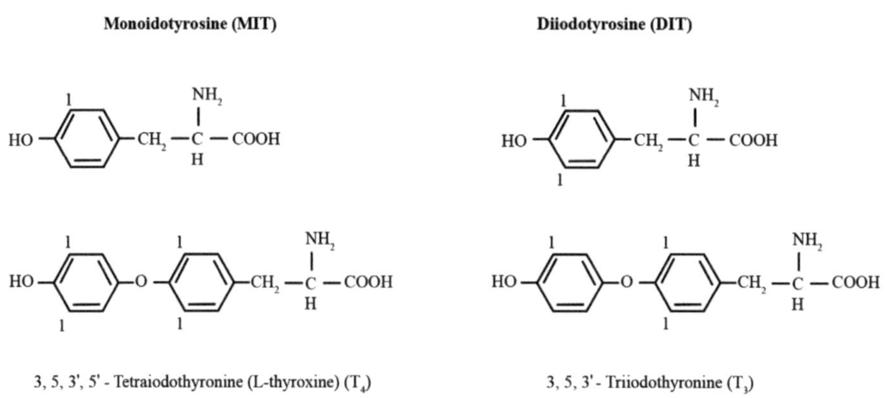

Figure 6.
Biochemical structure of T_3 and T_4 [26].

5. Thyroid hormones' physiological effects

- Intensify the basal metabolic rate.
- Na^+/K^+ ATPase synthesis should be encouraged.
- The rise in body temperature.
- Help in protein synthesis.
- Use more fatty acids and glucose to produce more ATP.
- Induce lipolysis.
- Regulate development and growth of nervous tissue and bones.

6. Autoimmune thyroid disease (AITD)

AITD is a complex and multifactorial disease in which the immune system attacks the thyroid gland by producing antibodies against thyroid antigens developed against a particular genetic background initiated by exposure to environmental factors. It is the most common endocrinal disease that occurs due to the formation of autoantibodies against thyroid-specific peroxidase and other receptor proteins, such as the thyrotropin receptor, present on thyrocytes [27]. These endocrinal diseases are characterized by the presence of antibodies such as TPO-Abs (thyroperoxidase antibodies) and thyroglobulin, produced by our own body system.

Silva et al. conducted a study of 89 Brazilian women, and they found that 90% of people with autoimmune thyroiditis have elevated anti-TPO [28]. Anti-TPO antibody was used more extensively by Lock et al. for clinical evaluation in subclinical hypothyroidism [29]. TPO antibody-positive people were found to be 13.3% in a study conducted in Delhi between 2007 and 2010 [30]. Similarly, an apparent increase in occurrence was observed in southern India. In two separate studies conducted in Kerala and Punjab, the comparable prevalence of anti-TPO positives was 16.7 and 36.5%, respectively [31, 32]. Jeena et al. reported that anti-TPO antibody estimates are useful in identifying the etiology of autoimmune thyroiditis. In that study, anti-TPO antibody titers were found to be elevated in 47 to 60% of patients with hypothyroidism [33].

7. Historical background of AITD

Hashimoto characterized hypothyroidism and goiter as a result of thyroid lymphoid invasion in 1912. Anti-Tg (antithyroglobulin) antibodies were discovered in similar patients in 1956, revealing the autoimmune origin of these traits, and activating TSH receptor antibodies were discovered at the same period of time. Anti-TPO antibodies were first identified as thyroid microsomal antibodies in 1964 but were later renamed anti-TPO because of their auto-antigen identity [34].

8. Epidemiology of AITD

AITD is considered the prototypical and most prevalent organ-specific endocrinal disease, affecting 2–5% of the iodine-sufficient population [35]. The first pathological features of AITD were described in 1912, when patients with goiter caused diffusion of lymphocyte infiltration and thyroid cellular atrophy in the clinical histological picture of thyroid tissue [36]. The incidence rate is 0.3–1.5 per 1000 persons per year, and it is 4–10 times higher in women than in men [2, 37, 38].

AITD is an organ-specific autoimmune disorder that is much more common in women than in men. About 1% of men are affected by this disease, whereas 2–4% women are suffering from it worldwide and with the advanced age, this trend is greater. In the USA and Canada, the prevalence rates are 5,873,102 and 6, 50,157, respectively. In China and India, the prevalence rates are 25, 976, 952 and 21,301,112, respectively. The annual incidence of Hashimoto's thyroiditis is believed to be 0.3–1.5 cases per 1000 people worldwide, while Grave's disease is expected to have five occurrences per 10,000 people. About 90% of AITDs are caused by Hashimoto's thyroiditis [39].

9. Etiological factors of AITD

As AITD is a multifactorial disease, the factors responsible for the initiation of AITD are mostly genetic, in which gene alteration occurs. Hormonal changes in females, medication adverse effects, smoking, aging, and iodine overconsumption are other endogenous and environmental factors that cause autoimmune thyroid disease [3, 4]. Environmental factors such as smoking, alcohol, iodine, stress, infections, and drugs are secondary etiological factors responsible for AITD. Female sex and parity are considered existential factors responsible for AITD because of certain sex hormonal imbalances, women are considered to be more prone to AITD as compared to men. Increased age has also been shown to be conclusively linked to AITD [40–44]. Certain gene alterations, such as TSH receptor, thyroglobulin, HLA, interleukins, and cytotoxic lymphocyte genes, are primary etiological factors responsible for causing AITD.

10. Pathophysiology of AITD

More than 30% of all organ-specific autoimmunity diseases are represented by thyroid autoimmune. About 3% of the population is affected by Hashimoto's thyroiditis, the earliest and most prevalent organ-specific autoimmune disease. It serves as the prototypical T-cell-mediated degenerative disease among others such as multiple sclerosis and type 1 diabetes [45–47]. However, the theory of cytotoxic T lymphocyte (CTL)-mediated target destruction in thyroid autoimmunity has lately been challenged [48–51]. A new theory of autoimmune target destruction in Hashimoto's thyroiditis has been developed as a result of advancements in the study of apoptosis and investigations of Graves' disease, a non-destructive type of thyroid autoimmunity.

It is thought that the thyroid antigen-specific CD4 (helper) T lymphocytes are what triggers the autoimmune thyroid disease process. T cells with this antigen-specificity have been isolated from the thyroid tissue of Grave's disease patients [47, 52].

Through the induction of activated T cells and subsequent production of gamma interferon, thyroid cells express MHC class II, which activates T-cell reticulation and sustains the autoimmune process [53, 54].

Since the thyroid itself encourages further expansion of the pertinent population of T cells; the mechanism underlying the initial activation of T cells may be less antigen-specific than in molecular mimicry. Self-reactive CD4 T cells promote autoreactive B cells to enter the thyroid and secrete thyroid antibodies. Thyroglobulin, the storage protein for thyroid hormones, thyroperoxidase, and TSH receptors are the three main target antigens for thyroid autoantibodies. In autoimmune thyroiditis, Th1, Th2, and Th17 immune responses involve active participation. Antigen-presenting cells and CD4+ T helper cells play a role in the activation of effector T cells, and as a result, thyroid-specific antigens (TPO and Tg) CD8+ T cells are activated, which proliferate cytotoxic T lymphocytes (CTL) that destroy thyroid cells, and on the other hand, B cells might develop into plasma cells, generating thyroid-restricted antibodies, followed by antibody- or complement-restricted thyroid cell death. It is believed that Th17 cells are also involved in the destruction process. Increase the release of thyroid-specific antigens by the destroyed thyrocytes, which leads to an acceleration of the immune process. Inhibition of regulatory T cells (Treg) as well as secretion of inflammatory molecules (CXCL8, CXCL10, and interferon-g) by the thyroid itself could further enhance the autoimmune process [55, 56] CD8 (cytotoxic) T cells and B cells are drawn into the thyroid by activated CD4 T cells [57, 58]. It is thought that the primary mechanism causing hypothyroidism involves CD8 cells directly killing thyroid cells. Thyroid autoantibodies, however, might also play a pathogenic role [59].

11. Types of autoimmune thyroid diseases

There are the following types of autoimmune thyroid disease:

1. Hashimoto's autoimmune thyroiditis (AITD), is atrophic and causes primary myxedema.

2. Grave's disease hyperthyroidism.

3. Postpartum thyroiditis (PPT).

4. Thyroid-associated orbitopathy (TAO).

In Graves' disease, thyroid-stimulating antibodies were found in 1956, and in 1957, thyroid antibodies were found in Hashimoto's disease [60, 61]. Hypertrophic thyroiditis is the most prevalent autoimmune thyroid disease in Hashimoto's disease. The immune system responds against the body's own tissue and it show features such as diffuse goiter, lymphocytic infiltration in the presence of autoantibody, and the gradual degeneration of the follicular cells of thyroid gland resulting in a deficiency of thyroid hormones, which help in the diagnosis of Hashimoto's thyroiditis [55, 57, 62]. Autoimmune thyroid disease results in two opposite pathogenic effects: hyperthyroidism in Grave's disease and thyroid destruction in Hashimoto's thyroiditis.

Hashimoto's thyroiditis is caused by self-reactive CD4+ T cells attracting B cells and CD8+ T cells to the thyroid. Thyroid cell death and hypothyroidism are symptoms of disease progression. It has been suggested that autoimmune thyrocyte depletion is caused by both autoantibodies and thyroid-specific cytotoxic T lymphocytes (CTLs). In Grave's disease, B cells release thyroid-stimulating immunoglobulins (TSI) against the thyroid-stimulating hormone receptor (TSHR), which is triggered by activated CD4+ T cells. This results in hyperthyroidism and unregulated thyroid hormone production [63].

Grave's disease is characterized by elevated levels of thyroid-specific autoantibodies and circulating activated T cells. These anti-TSH receptor antibodies promote thyroid activity and cause hyperactivity of the gland [61]. While free T_3 and free T_4 hormone concentrations are within the normal range, subclinical Hashimoto's thyroiditis is identified by a decreased serum TSH level (less than 0.3 mIU/ml). TSH and thyroid hormone levels are both decreased in clinically present (Over) hypothyroidism [64]. In Grave's disease, hyperthyroidism occurs, which leads to enlargement of the thyroid gland. In the case of Grave's disease, anti-TPO antibodies do not play a major role but majorly cause Hashimoto's thyroidism.

It is common to have subclinical hypothyroidism. The prevalence ranges from 3 to 8%, rising with age and affecting more women than men. Around 10% of men and women experience combined prevalence after the sixth decade. Anti-thyroid antibodies are present in 80% of these patients, and 80% of them have serum TSH levels that are less than 10 mIU/L [65]. Although a patient with subclinical hypothyroidism does not exhibit the appropriate signs and symptoms, there is a slight increase in TSH and anti-TPO levels, which are still within normal ranges for free T_3 and free T_4 levels.

About 2 to 5 percent of cases per year will progress from subclinical hypothyroidism to overt hypothyroidism. Early diagnosis and treatment help prevent the onset of overt hypothyroidism and its negative effects on the body's system because subclinical hypothyroidism is more common than overt hypothyroidism [66]. High anti-TPO patient titers increase the risk of overt condition changes and increase symptom severity.

According to the National Health and Nutrition Examination Survey III (NHANES), over 10 percent of adults tested positive for either TPO-Ab or Tg-Ab, with a prevalence of 13% for TPO-Ab and 11.5% for Tg-Ab [67]. In a study conducted by Atieh Amouzegar et al., out of 5783 participants, 742 (12.8%) tested positive for TPO-Ab, with women more likely than men to do so. In the general population, TPO-Ab positivity was present in 11.9, 14.9, and 13.6% of the young, middle-aged, and elderly, respectively [68].

12. TPO introduction and role in body

TPO, previously known as thyroid microsomal antigen, was defined in 1985, responsible for the autoimmune response in AITD [69]. It is an enzyme that is present in microsomes of thyrocytes and expressed on the apical surface of thyroid cells. Thyroperoxidase is also called thyroid-specific peroxidases, as it is only present in thyrocytes and not in any other organ of the body. The secreted recombinant human TPO comprises 842 amino acids and has a predicted molecular mass of 93.8 kDa [70].

TPO plays a key enzyme role in the biosynthesis of thyroid hormone. This process takes place in thyrocytes at the apical membrane colloid interface and requires thyroglobulin, iodine, and hydrogen peroxide. Iodide is actively transported into the follicular cells through the sodium iodide support system. In follicular cells, the process of deiodination occurs when iodine is used to create the active ionic form of iodide. TPO oxidizes iodide by using hydrogen peroxide created in the cell's peroxisomes, which cause

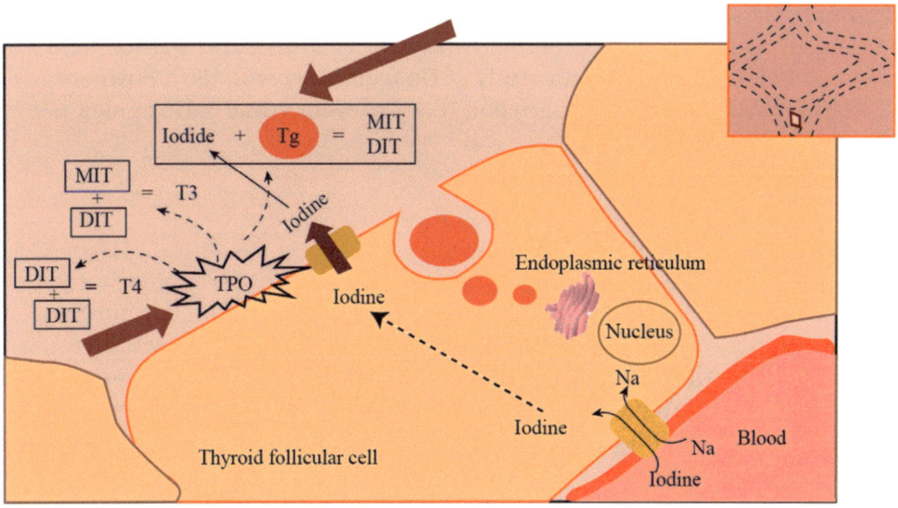

Figure 7.
Function of Thyroperoxidase in thyrocytes, coupling of MIT and DIT, synthesis of T3 and T4 [71].

covalent bonds to form with the thyroglobulin residue, that is, tyrosyl. MIT (monoiodotyrosine) and DIT (di- iodotyrosine) are produced as a result. Two DIT combine to form T_4 (thyroxine) and one MIT and one DIT combine to form T_3 (tri-Iodothyronine), which is illustrated in **Figure 7** [71]. The coupling reaction is also catalyzed by TPO in the presence of hydrogen peroxidase [72]. So, in addition to working in concert with thyroglobulin, the TPO enzyme is crucial for the iodination of L-tyrosine and the chemical coupling of mono- and di-iodotyrosine to produce thyroid hormones [5, 73].

13. Role of TPO antibodies in AITD (autoimmune thyroid disease)

In cases of autoimmune thyroid disorders, the body's autoantibodies start to produce antibodies against the thyroperoxidase enzyme, called as anti-thyroperoxidase antibodies [74]. These antibodies mistakenly attack normal tissue, such as thyrocytes in the thyroid gland. Due to the attack of anti-TPO antibodies, there is inflammation and impaired function of the thyroid gland [75]. Several studies report that antibody-dependent cell-mediated cytotoxicity could be induced by thyroperoxidase antibodies. TPO-Ab is frequently found in the general population and has more specificity than other antibodies; this antibody directly involves thyroid cellular damage and is positively correlated with the activity of chronic thyroiditis [76]. Autoantibodies to TPO are more common in the euthyroid population. Elevated serum titers of antibodies to TPO are found in several forms of thyroiditis caused by autoimmune disorders [77]. Inflammation or destruction of the thyroid gland, like in Hashimoto's disease, may be indicated by the presence of TPO antibodies. Whereas other forms of thyroiditis, such as postpartum thyroid dysfunction (PPTD), are less commonly associated with TPO antibodies [78].

Anti-TPO antibodies are more sensitive in diagnosing thyroid autoimmune diseases. Some patients have mildly elevated levels of anti-TPO antibodies but do not show sign or symptoms. The presence of TPO antibodies increases the risk of future thyroid disorders. In such patients, the doctor recommends periodic checkups to monitor the prognosis of thyroid ailments.

In the HUNT study, positive TPO-Ab was found in 2.8% of men and 13.9% of women, aged over 40 years [79]. Similarly positive TPO-Ab status was found in 8.6% of men and 18.5% of women in the study of Hoogendoorn et al. [80]. Furthermore, TPO-Ab titers >200 kU/l were reported in 16.9% of women and 6.6% of men in a study conducted in Denmark [81].

14. Signs and symptoms of AITD

Signs and symptoms of autoimmune thyroid disease depend on thyroid gland function, whether the patient is suffering from hyperthyroidism or hypothyroidism. In the case of hyperthyroidism, the symptoms will be sweating, rapid heart rate, tremors, weight loss, fatigue, anxiety, sleeping difficulty, etc. In the case of hypothyroidism, symptoms will include weight gain, dry skin, hair loss, cold intolerance, constipation, fatigue, etc. The signs and symptoms will vary as per the severity of the disease, which is illustrated in **Table 2**. This could be permanent if AITD is at a chronic stage. Symptoms may come and go depending on whether the person receives treatment, and whether the treatment takes effect.

15. Laboratory diagnosis of AITD

For laboratory diagnosis, the doctor recommends thyroid function testing along with thyroid antibody testing. In a thyroid function test, the following parameters are checked:

- TSH (Thyroid-stimulating hormone) testing.
- Free T_3 (Tri-iodotyrosine)
- Free T_4 (Tetra-iodotyrosine)
- Anti TPO Ab testing.

Hyperthyroidism: Increased T_3 and T_4	Hypothyroidism: Decreased T_3 and T_4
Increased basal metabolic rate	Decreased BMR
Anxiety, physical restlessness, mental excitability	Depression, psychosis, mental slowness, lethargy
Hair loss	Dry and brittle hair
Tachycardia, palpitation and fibrillation	Bradycardia
Diarrhea	Constipation
Weight loss and good appetite	Weight gain, anorexia
Warm sweaty skin, heat intolerance	Dry cold skin, prone to hypothermia

Table 2.
Common sign and symptoms in hyperthyroidism and hypothyroidism.

Free T_3 and free T_4 are both biologically active forms, and they are free in circulation, so their value remains constant and is not affected by the concentration of circulatory proteins. So, free T_3 and free T_4 are preferred over total T_3 and T_4.

In thyroid antibody testing, TG antibodies and TPO antibodies are determined, as these are commonly found autoantibodies that are frequently present in serum. Anti-TPO is more sensitive and has more specificity for the diagnosis of thyroid autoimmune disease and hence is preferred.

16. Normal reference values

The following **Table 3** shows the reference range of thyroid parameters:

17. Interpretations

Subclinical hypothyroidism occurs when patients have no signs or symptoms as such, mildly elevated values of anti-TPO antibodies and TSH, but normal levels of other thyroid hormones such as free T_3 and free T_4. If subclinical thyroid is left untreated for a long time, it can switch over to an overt hypothyroidism condition, and the patient becomes symptomatic. In overt hypothyroidism, the levels of anti-TPO antibody titer and TSH are markedly elevated, along with mildly variably elevated levels of other thyroid hormones, such as free T_3 and free T_4.

18. Role of TPO-Ab in disease pathogenesis

TPO-Ab is uncommon in healthy children and adolescent is low, but the prevalence increases with age and especially predominant in females [32, 82]. Anti-TPOs are detected mostly in patients with autoimmune hypothyroidism. The presence of TPO-Ab contributes to the confirmation of the autoimmune nature of thyroid failure. In patients with "borderline" thyroid function test, TPO-Ab status can be used for treatment decisions. Furthermore, even in people with normal TSH and thyroid hormone levels, the presence of TPO-Ab, particularly in younger age groups, can predict the development of future thyroid dysfunction. Evidence suggests that antibody status can determine the clinical course of autoimmune hypothyroidism.

Parameter	Normal range
Anti-TPO (Thyroperoxidase) U/ml	5.0–35.0
TSH (uIU/ml)	0.27–4.20
Free T_3 (pg/ml)	2.0–4.4
Free T_4 (ng/dl)	0.93–1.73

Table 3.
Normal reference ranges of thyroid function test for ATD diagnosis.

19. Conclusion

This organ-specific endocrinal disease is becoming a major and challenging disease worldwide. Autoimmune thyroid diseases occur due to immune-mediated alterations in the thyroid gland, which produce functional alterations in thyroid hormone status. Proper diagnosis helps with better treatment of this disease.

Thyroid hormone synthesis significantly relies on the TPO enzyme. In order to diagnose autoimmune thyroid disease and forecast its clinical course, measuring the levels of anti-TPO autoantibodies has been reported to be important. In order to identify the cause of hypothyroidism and the likelihood that a patient's subclinical condition will progress to overt hypothyroidism, serum TSH and anti-TPO analyses are crucial. TSH, free T_3, and free T_4 levels also aid in the diagnosis of autoimmune thyroid disease and help distinguish between overt and subclinical hypothyroidism.

Acknowledgements

I would like to thank Jasjot Singh for his help in writing, and I would also like to thank Asso. Prof. Pitambar Lamichane and Resham Shrestha for their help in drawing. I am eternally grateful to all of you for this.

Conflict of interest

The author declares no conflict of interest.

Abbreviations

AIDS	acquired immunodeficiency syndrome
AITD	autoimmune thyroid disease
Anti-Tg	anti-thyroglobulin
APCs	antigen presenting cells
ATP	amino triphosphate
CLT	cytotoxic T lymphocyte
DIT	di-iodotyrosine
HIV	human immunodeficiency virus
HLA	human leucocyte antigen
LPS	lipopolysaccharides
MHC	major histocompatibility complex
MIT	mono-iodotyrosine
NHANES	National health and nutrition examination survey III
PAMPs	pathogens that have similar molecular patterns
PPT	postpartum thyroiditis
PPTD	postpartum thyroid dysfunction
PRR	pattern recognition receptors
RNA	ribonucleic acid
TAO	thyroid-associated orbitopathy
TCR T	cell receptor
Tg	thyroglobulin

DOI: http://dx.doi.org/10.5772/intechopen.1004070

TPO	thyroperoxidase
TPO-Abs	thyroperoxidase antibodies
TSH	thyroid stimulating hormone
T3	tri-iodotyrosine
T4	tetra-iodotyrosine

Author details

Nurakant Neupane
National Academy of Medical Sciences, Bir Hospital, Kathmandu, Nepal

*Address all correspondence to: nurakantn@gmail.com

References

[1] Swain M, Swain T, Mohanty BK. Autoimmune thyroid disorders-an update. Indian Journal of Clinical Biochemistry. 2005;**20**(1):9-17

[2] Canaris GJ, Manowitz NR, Mayor G, Ridgway EC. The colorado thyroid disease prevalence study. Archives of Internal Medicine. 2000;**160**(4):526-534

[3] Holt PG. Immune and inflammatory function in cigarette smokers. Thorax. 1987;**42**(4):241-249

[4] Nelson JLSA. In: Berczi IKK, editor. Sex Steroids, Autoimmunity and Autoimmune Disease. London, Lancaster: MTP Press; 1987. pp. 93-119

[5] Gey A, Diallo A, Seneschal J, Léauté-Labrèze C, Boralevi F, Jouary T, et al. Autoimmune thyroid disease in vitiligo: Multivariate analysis indicates intricate pathomechanisms. The British Journal of Dermatology. 2013;**168**(4):756-761

[6] Turnbridge WMG, Evered DC, Hall R, Appleton D, Brewis M, Clark F, et al. The spectrum of thyroid disease in a community: The whickham survey. Clinical Endocrinology. 1977;7:481-493. DOI: 10.1111/j.1365-2265.1977.tb01340.x

[7] Parham P, Janeway C. The Immune System. 5th ed. New York: Garland Science, Taylor & Francis; 2021

[8] Alberts B, Heald R, Johnson A, Morgan DO, Raff MC, Roberts K, et al. Molecular Biology of the Cell. 7th ed. New York: W. W. Norton & Company; 2022

[9] Bonilla FA, Oettgen HC. Adaptive immunity. The Journal of Allergy and Clinical Immunology. 2010;**125** (2 Suppl. 2):S33-S40

[10] Marshall JS, Warrington R, Watson W, Kim HL. An introduction to immunology and immunopathology. Allergy, Asthma & Clinical Immunology. 2018;**14**(2):49

[11] Murphy K, Weaver C. Janeway's Immunobiology. 9th ed. New York: Garland science; 2016

[12] White AM. A Guide to Transfer Factors and Immune System Health. 2nd ed. North Chasleston, SC: BookSurge; 2009

[13] Gell PGH, Coombs RRA. Clinical Aspects of Immunology. Philadelphia: Davis; 1963

[14] Rajan TV. The Gell-Coombs classification of hypersensitivity reactions: A re-interpretation. Trends in Immunology. 2003;**24**(7):376-379

[15] Notarangelo LD. Primary immunodeficiencies. The Journal of Allergy and Clinical Immunology. 2010;**125**(2 Suppl. 2):S182-S194

[16] Chinen J, Shearer WT. Secondary immunodeficiencies, including HIV infection. The Journal of Allergy and Clinical Immunology. 2010;**125** (2 Suppl. 2):S195-S203

[17] Sinha AA, Lopez MT, McDevitt HO. Autoimmune diseases: The failure of self tolerance. Science. 1990;**248**(4961):1380-1388

[18] Castro C, Gourley M. Diagnostic testing and interpretation of tests for autoimmunity. The Journal of Allergy and Clinical Immunology. 2010;**125** (2 Suppl. 2):S238-S247

[19] Gley E. Sur les fonctions du corps thyroid. Comptes rendus des séances de

la societe de biologie et de ses Filiales. 1891;**43**:841-842

[20] Graves RJ. Newly observed affection of the thyroid gland in females. Medical-Surgical Nursing Journal. 1835;7:516

[21] Jr HR. Thyroid and antithyroid drugs. In: Gilman AG, Rall TW, Nies AS, et al., editors. The Pharmacological Basis of Therapeutics. 8th ed. New York: Pergamon Press; 1990. pp. 1361-1383

[22] Vanderpump MPJ, Tunbridge WMG. Epidemiology and prevention of clinical and subclinical hypothyroidism. Thyroid. 2002;**12**(10):839-847

[23] Wiersinga WM. Subclinical hypothyroidism and hyperthyroidism. I. Prevalence and clinical relevance. The Netherlands Journal of Medicine. 1995;**46**(4):197-204

[24] Available from: https://www.kegg.jp/entry/map04918

[25] Tortora GJ, Derrickson BH. Principles of Anatomy and Physiology [Internet]. 12th ed. Philadelphia: John Wiley & Sons; 2008. Available from: https://books.google.com.np/books?id=uNwfOPPYgKAC

[26] Satyanarayana U, Chakrapani U. Biochemistry. 6th ed. New Delhi: Elsevier; 2021

[27] McIntosh RS, Asghar MS, Weetman AP. The antibody response in human autoimmune thyroid disease. Clinical Science. 1997;**92**:529-541

[28] Silva LM, Chavez J, Canalli MHB, Zanetti CR. Determination of IgG subclasses and avidity of antithyroid peroxidase antibodies in patients with subclinical hypothyroidism - a comparison with patients with overt hypothyroidism. Hormone Research. 2003;**59**(3):118-124

[29] Lock RJ, Marden NA, Kemp HJ, Thomas PH, Goldie DJ, Gompels MM. Subclinical hypothyroidism: A comparison of strategies to achieve adherence to treatment guidelines. Annals of Clinical Biochemistry. 2004;**41**(Pt 3):197-200

[30] Unnikrishnan AG, Kalra S, Sahay RK, Bantwal G, John M, Tewari N. Prevalence of hypothyroidism in adults: An epidemiological study in eight cities of India. Indian Journal of Endocrinology and Metabolism. 2013;**17**(4):647-652

[31] Marwaha RK, Tandon N, Ganie MA, Kanwar R, Sastry A, Garg MK, et al. Status of thyroid function in Indian adults: Two decades after universal salt iodization. The Journal of the Association of Physicians of India. 2012;**60**:32-36

[32] Singh J, Prabhakar PK, Neupane N. Hospital-based clinical study on prevalence of TPO antibodies in association to autoimmune thyroid diseases in tertiary care hospital. Asian Journal of Pharmaceutical and Clinical Research [Internet]. 2020;**13**:186-189; Available from: https://api.semanticscholar.org/CorpusID:234539770

[33] Jeena E, Malathi M, Sudeep K. A hospital-based study of anti-TPO titer in patients with thyroid disease. Muller Journal of Medical Sciences and Research [Internet]. 2013;**4**(2):74-77. Available from: https://www.mjmsr.net/article.asp?issn=0975-9727

[34] Saravanan P, Dayan CM. Thyroid autoantibodies. Endocrinology and Metabolism Clinics of North America. 2001;**30**(2):315-337, viii

[35] Sgarbi JA, Maciel RMB. Pathogenesis of autoimmune thyroid diseases. Arquivos Brasileiros de Endocrinologia e Metabologia. 2009;**53**(1):5-14

[36] Hashimoto H. Zur Kenntniss der lymphomatosen Veranderung der Schilddruse (struma lymphomatosa). Arch Klin Chir. 1912;**97**(219):219-248

[37] Huber A, Menconi F, Corathers S, Jacobson EM, Tomer Y. Joint genetic susceptibility to type 1 diabetes and autoimmune thyroiditis: From epidemiology to mechanisms. Endocrine Reviews. 2008;**29**(6):697-725

[38] Iddah MA, Macharia BN, Ng'wena AG, Keter A, AVO O. Thryroid hormones and hematological indices levels in thyroid disorders patients at moi teaching and referral hospital, Western Kenya. ISRN Endocrinology. 2013;**2013**:385940

[39] Vanderpump MP, Tunbridge WM, French JM, Appleton D, Bates D, Clark F, et al. The incidence of thyroid disorders in the community: A twenty-year follow-up of the Whickham survey. Clinical Endocrinology. 1995;**43**(1):55-68

[40] Ghoraishian SM, Hekmati Moghaddam SH, Afkhami-Ardekani M. Relationship between anti-thyroid peroxidase antibody and thyroid function test. Iranian Journal of Immunology. 2006;**3**(3):146-149

[41] Nagataki S, Yamashita S, Tamai H. Immunogenetics of autoimmune endocrine disease. In: Volpe R, editor. Autoimmune Diseases of Endocrine System. Boca Raton: CRC Press; 1990. pp. 51-72

[42] Schleusener H, Bogner U, Peters H, Kotulla P, Schmieg D, Grüters A, et al. The relevance of genetic susceptibility in Graves' disease and immune thyroiditis. Experimental and Clinical Endocrinology. 1991;**97**(2-3):127-132

[43] Plotnikoff NP, Murgo AJ, Faith RE. Stress and Immunity [Internet]. Boca Raton: Taylor & Francis; 1991

[44] Glaser R, Kiecolt-Glaser JK. Handbook of Human Stress and Immunity. St Louis, Missouri, USA: Elsevier Science; 2014

[45] Wucherpfennig KW, Eisenbarth GS. Type 1 diabetes. Nature Immunology. 2001;**2**:767-768

[46] Steinman L. Multiple sclerosis: A two-stage disease. Nature Immunology. 2001;**2**:762-764

[47] Weetman AP, McGregor AM. Autoimmune thyroid disease: Further developments in our understanding. Endocrine Reviews. 1994;**15**(6):788-830

[48] Giordano C, Stassi G, De Maria R, Todaro M, Richiusa P, Papoff G, et al. Potential involvement of Fas and its ligand in the pathogenesis of Hashimoto's thyroiditis. Science. 1997;**275**(5302):960-963

[49] De Maria R, Testi R. Fas-FasL interactions: A common pathogenetic mechanism in organ-specific autoimmunity. Immunology Today. 1998;**19**(3):121-125

[50] Stassi G, Todaro M, Bucchieri F, Stoppacciaro A, Farina F, Zummo G, et al. Fas/Fas ligand-driven T cell apoptosis as a consequence of ineffective thyroid immunoprivilege in Hashimoto's thyroiditis. Journal of Immunology. 1999;**162**(1):263-267

[51] Stassi G, Di Liberto D, Todaro M, Zeuner A, Ricci-Vitiani L, Stoppacciaro A, et al. Control of target cell survival in thyroid autoimmunity by T helper cytokines via regulation of apoptotic proteins. Nature Immunology. 2000;**1**(6):483-488

[52] Bottazzo GF, Pujol-Borrell R, Hanafusa T, Feldmann M. Role of aberrant HLA-DR expression and antigen

presentation in induction of endocrine autoimmunity. Lancet (London, England). 1983;**2**(8359):1115-1119

[53] Londei M, Bottazzo GF, Feldmann M. Human T-cell clones from autoimmune thyroid glands: Specific recognition of autologous thyroid cells. Science. 1985;**228**(4695):85-89

[54] Dayan CM, Londei M, Corcoran AE, Grubeck-Loebenstein B, James RF, Rapoport B, et al. Autoantigen recognition by thyroid-infiltrating T cells in Graves disease. Proceedings of the National Academy of Sciences of the United States of America. 1991;**88**(16):7415-7419

[55] Mooij P, de Wit HJ, Bloot AM, Wilders-Truschnig MM, Drexhage HA. Iodine deficiency induces thyroid autoimmune reactivity in Wistar rats. Endocrinology. 1993;**133**(3):1197-1204

[56] Ehlers M, Schott M. Hashimoto's thyroiditis and papillary thyroid cancer: Are they immunologically linked? Trends in Endocrinology and Metabolism. 2014;**25**(12):656-664. DOI: 10.1016/j.tem.2014.09.001. Epub 2014 Oct 9

[57] Dayan CM, Daniels GH. Chronic autoimmune thyroiditis. The New England Journal of Medicine. 1996;**335**(2):99-107

[58] Schott M, Scherbaum WA. Autoimmune thyroid disease. Dtsch Arztebl. 2006;**103**(45):A3023-A3032

[59] Eguchi K. Apoptosis in autoimmune diseases. Internal Medicine. 2001;**40**(4):275-284

[60] Adams DD. Abnormal response in the assay of thyrotropin. Proceedings of the University of Otago Medical School. 1956;**34**:11-12

[61] Doniach D, Roitt IM. Autoimmunity in Hashimoto's disease and its implications. The Journal of Clinical Endocrinology and Metabolism. 1957;**17**(11):1293-1304

[62] Neupane N, Kaur M, Prabhakar PK. Treatment of Hashimoto's thyroiditis with herbal medication. International Journal of Green Pharmacy. 2017;**11**(3):S343- S347

[63] Stassi G, De Maria R. Autoimmune thyroid disease: New models of cell death in autoimmunity. Nature Reviews. Immunology. 2002;**2**:195-204. DOI: 10.1038/nri750

[64] Hueston WJ. Treatment of hypothyroidism. American Family Physician. 2001;**64**(10):1717-1724

[65] Fatourechi V. Subclinical hypothyroidism: An update for primary care physicians. Mayo Clinic Proceedings. 2009;**84**(1):65-71

[66] Cooper DS. Subclinical hypothyroidism. JAMA. 1987;**258**:246-247

[67] Pedersen IB, Knudsen N, Jørgensen T, Perrild H, Ovesen L, Laurberg P. Thyroid peroxidase and thyroglobulin autoantibodies in a large survey of populations with mild and moderate iodine deficiency. Clinical Endocrinology. 2003;**58**(1):36-42

[68] Amouzegar A, Gharibzadeh S, Kazemian E, Mehran L, Tohidi M, Azizi F. The prevalence, incidence and natural course of positive antithyroperoxidase antibodies in a population-based study: Tehran thyroid study. PLoS One. 2017;**12**(1):e0169283

[69] Czarnocka B, Ruf J, Ferrand M, Carayon P, Lissitzky S. Purification of the human thyroid peroxidase and its identification as the microsomal antigen

involved in autoimmune thyroid diseases. FEBS Letters. 1985;**190**(1):147-152

[70] Ruf J, Carayon P. Structural and functional aspects of thyroid peroxidase. Archives of Biochemistry and Biophysics. 2006;**445**(2):269-277

[71] Balucan FS, Morshed SA, Davies TF. Thyroid autoantibodies in pregnancy: Their role, regulation and clinical relevance. Journal of Thyroid Research. 2013;**2013**:182472, 15 pages. DOI: 10.1155/2013/182472

[72] Song Y, Driessens N, Costa M, De Deken X, Detours V, Corvilain B, et al. Roles of hydrogen peroxide in thyroid physiology and disease. The Journal of Clinical Endocrinology and Metabolism. 2007;**92**(10):3764-3773

[73] Il SJ, Kim MJ, Lee JS. Graves' disease, rheumatoid arthritis, and anti-tumor necrosis factor-alpha therapy. The Journal of Rheumatology. 2009;**36**:449-450; author reply 450

[74] Volpe R. Autoimmune Diseases of the Endocrine System. Boca Raton: CRC Press, Taylor & Francis; 1990. ISBN: 9780849368493

[75] Beever K, Bradbury J, Phillips D, McLachlan SM, Pegg C, Goral A, et al. Highly sensitive assays of autoantibodies to thyroglobulin and to thyroid peroxidase. Clinical Chemistry. 1989;**35**(9):1949-1954

[76] Li Y, Teng D, Shan Z, Teng X, Guan H, Yu X, et al. Antithyroperoxidase and antithyroglobulin antibodies in a five-year follow-up survey of populations with different iodine intakes. The Journal of Clinical Endocrinology and Metabolism. 2008;**93**(5):1751-1757

[77] Pfannenstiel P, Hotze LSBS. Schilddrüsenkrankheiten Diagnose und Therapie. 2nd ed. Berlin: Berliner Medizinische Verlagsanstalt; 1995. pp. 28-30, 141, 169 – 172, 200 – 201 p

[78] Swelam EESA, Bakr HG, Mansour MAE-A. Postpartum thyroid dysfunction: A state of immunological dysregulation. Clinical Laboratory. 2011;**57**(9-10):731-739

[79] Bjoro T, Holmen J, Krüger O, Midthjell K, Hunstad K, Schreiner T, et al. Prevalence of thyroid disease, thyroid dysfunction and thyroid peroxidase antibodies in a large, unselected population. The health study of Nord-Trondelag (HUNT). European Journal of Endocrinology. 2000;**143**(5):639-647

[80] Hoogendoorn EH, Hermus AR, de Vegt F, Ross HA, Verbeek ALM, Kiemeney LALM, et al. Thyroid function and prevalence of anti-thyroperoxidase antibodies in a population with borderline sufficient iodine intake: Influences of age and sex. Clinical Chemistry. 2006;**52**(1):104-111

[81] Knudsen N, Jorgensen T, Rasmussen S, Christiansen E, Perrild H. The prevalence of thyroid dysfunction in a population with borderline iodine deficiency. Clinical Endocrinology. 1999;**51**(3):361-367

[82] Roti E, Gardini E, Minelli R, Bianconi L, Braverman LE. Prevalence of anti-thyroid peroxidase antibodies in serum in the elderly: Comparison with other tests for anti-thyroid antibodies. Clinical Chemistry. 1992;**38**(1):88-92